FIRMING
YOUR
FIGURE

HAMLYN HELP YOURSELF GUIDE

FIRMING YOUR FIGURE

HELEN DORE

HAMLYN

First published in 1990 by
The Hamlyn Publishing Group Limited,
a division of the Octopus Publishing Group,
Michelin House, 81 Fulham Road,
London SW3 6RB

Copyright © The Hamlyn Publishing Group Limited

ISBN 0 600 57068 1

Typeset by SX Composing Ltd, Rayleigh, Essex
Printed and bound in Great Britain by Collins, Glasgow

Contents

ONE

Firm Facts

A firm figure is undoubtedly one of life's great assets, but by no means necessarily one of life's lucky draws! For most of us, it is something that has to be worked hard for, and once acquired, maintained with a similar degree of effort. Which is why a firm figure is something of which you can be justifiably proud: you look good and you feel good, knowing that you have done, and are continuing to do, the very best for both your appearance and your health.

Firming your figure doesn't just result in more attractive, visually appealing contours, and looking smarter in swimsuits, shorts, jeans, pencil-slim skirts and other figure-enhancing clothes – as tight and as bright as you like! It also means good posture and bearing, and an abundance of energy, all reflected in how you feel about yourself, how you relate to other people, and how you live your life generally.

A firm, lithe body does wonders for your self-esteem, and the sense of control and extra confidence it gives you in the way you feel about yourself means that you project a positive, attractive image which will stand you in good stead in both your work and your social life. There's no doubt about it – we are so often judged on the way we look, in all kinds of situations, from a job interview to meeting new people at a party. So if your appearance is trim and streamlined, then there is every likelihood that you will come across as an energetic, vital and dynamic, yet relaxed, personality – useful and fun to have around.

If you are reading this book the chances are that you are not 100 per cent happy about the state of your body, in which case you are in good company – the majority of people are self-critical about the way they look figure-wise. The good news is that exchanging a flabby figure for a firm one is within everyone's reach, irrespective of body type, age and sex – and you don't have to be a fitness fanatic, let alone a body-builder, either!

Diet and exercise

There's no mystique about firming your body to achieve a sleek, svelte and supple silhouette. It's basically achieved in two ways:

■ Eliminating excess body fat by eating the right kind of food, in the right balance to supply your body with all the nutrients it needs, in the right quantities to meet your energy requirements and no more.

■ Toning and conditioning the muscles, to make them strong, flexible and resilient, by doing the right kind of exercise on such a regular basis that it becomes as much part of your everyday life as eating or sleeping.

Diet and exercise should not be regarded as alternatives, or as mutually exclusive: the quickest and most effective way to achieve – and, most importantly, keep – the firm figure of your dreams is by combining them. You will lose weight by following a sensible, balanced diet, and if you follow the diet advice given in Chapter 8, the weight will stay off. But losing weight in itself does not necessarily automatically involve getting firm. If you lose a lot of weight, your figure may still re-

8

main slack, and the body does not always shed weight uniformly and evenly. It may fall off your hips, thighs and bust, for example, but your tummy – for many people a major problem and prime target area – may remain stubbornly prominent and disappointingly slack.

Exercise can be of tremendous help in such a situation. Although there is no such thing as a 'spot-reducing' exercise, 'spot-toning' exercises, working on specific body areas, can work wonders. (You'll find suggestions for these in Chapter 4.) As the exercising muscles draw on the surrounding fat, so the unsightly deposits diminish, and firmer, tauter muscles become more visible. And, of course, if you are dieting as well, to get rid of the fat covering the muscles which you are exercising, the results will show that much quicker. You will also be able to enjoy a much wider range of exercise, with less danger of strain or injury.

Incidentally, once you get established in a diet-and-exercise routine, don't be surprised if the scales don't always show as positive a loss as the tape measure. Muscles expand as they are worked, and healthy, well-exercised muscle tissue, which is denser than fat, weighs significantly more than when the muscles are shrunk through under-use. This is why the charts that show ideal weight as a function of height can be misleading. Not only can they fail to take body type and frame size into account but they also cannot distinguish between the weight of undesirable excess fat, and the weight of healthy, highly desirable, muscle mass.

Facing facts

Once you have decided to embark on getting your figure into better shape – and taking this initial decision in a committed way is absolutely crucial to success, as the next chapter explains in detail – then the very best thing you can do to start off with is to take a close, objective look at what you eat, and the amount of exercise you normally take. Ask yourself some really frank questions, and be perfectly honest with your answers!

A good way of going about this is to keep notes over a whole week of exactly what you eat and drink every day, going into as much detail as possible. Don't omit those between-meal snacks, if you've indulged in them! At the same time, note down how far you have walked and for how long, sports you have played, and conscious exercise you have taken.

If you are carrying an excess of body fat, then the chances are that your notes will tell you that your consumption of fat – especially saturated fat, the kind of animal fat you find in red meat, butter, cream, Cheddar cheese, for example – is too high. The same is likely to be true of refined sugar, present in great quantities not only in sweets, cakes, biscuits, ice-cream, etc., but in foods where you might be less likely to expect it – some convenience foods such as tinned cream soups, for example, and wine and spirits. And if you are also in the habit of eating a lot of fried food and junk foods, like potato chips, crisps, and other savoury commercial snacks, then you have already gone a long way towards explaining why you have good reason to be dissatisfied with your figure.

The conclusion you must draw is that your calorie intake is greater than your calorie expenditure. Fatty and sugary foods are notoriously high in calories – 1 gram of fat, for example, contains 9 calories, more than twice as many as 1 gram of complex carbohydrate or protein. Sugary foods, in particular, supply what are sometimes called 'empty' calories. This means that they do not provide valuable nutrients of the kind found in foods which are sources of complex carbohydrate, vitamins and minerals, such as fresh fruit and vegetables, cereals, grains and pulses, or in lean meat, chicken (without the skin) and fish, which provide body-building protein with a minimum of fat.

When you are taking in more calories through your food than you need for your energy requirements, the excess, instead of being converted into energy, is stored as fat deposits in the body. One way you can rectify this is to reduce the number of calories you consume, to bring intake and output, consumption and expenditure, into balance. Another is to develop a more active lifestyle, taking more exercise to use up more calories. Exercising regularly will increase your metabolic rate – the rate at which food is converted into energy and consumed – and eventually your body will continue to burn up extra calories even when it is at rest – for as long as 24 hours after vigorous sustained exercise. This is just one of the reasons why exercise is now generally acknowledged to have a key role to play in preventing disease and maintaining health.

Your figure and your health

It is quite possible that the fact-finding notes you have made indicate that you have taken no significant exercise at all in the course of the recorded week. If so, you are not alone. The increasingly sedentary lifestyle involving sometimes absolutely minimal physical effort, which far too many people have come to lead in the course of this century, is today regarded as a major health hazard. It is as much of a problem as eating the wrong diet, suffering from stress, or even smoking. About 40 per cent of adults in the UK are overweight, and alarmingly increased numbers of children are becoming so.

The miracle of the new technology can indeed be seen to have its dark side in health terms if you consider how easy it is to drive rather than walk; to take a lift or escalator rather than use the stairs; to make full use of the wealth of time- and labour-saving devices now available to us all at both home and work.

It is useful to bear in mind the minimal amount of progressive, vigorous exercise which experts advise as a basic requirement for keeping your body in adequate working order. This works out at 20-30 minutes at least three times a week – a total of about 1½ hours, which is really not very much when you consider that most of us spend more than 50 hours a week asleep, and many of us 20 hours or more watching TV!

Eating an excess of fatty, refined foods at the expense of natural wholefoods, can result among other things in dangerously high levels in the blood of cholesterol, an important component of the blood fats (lipoids), which have been strongly associated with heart disease. Taking too little exercise results in weakened muscles and an impaired cardiovascular system – a less efficiently working heart and lungs. Together, these have emerged as two of the most significantly contributory factors to the biggest silent killer of 20th-century Western society – coronary disease. More than 200,000 people in the UK alone (i.e. a quarter of the country's overall mortality rate) fall victim every year to a fatal heart attack.

Counterbalancing this depressing statistic is the fact that so much more knowledge is now available about what we can all do to create a healthier lifestyle for ourselves – in particular, by revising our eating and exercising habits. So even if your decision to set about firming your figure is primarily for aesthetic reasons – because you want to look good – you can be equally sure that in general health terms you will be doing yourself a tremendous favour, and giving your body the very least it deserves.

FAT FACTS

No more than 10-15% of the body's weight should consist of fat. But in the West, in the case of people leading a predominantly sedentary existence, the proportion is more likely to be 25-35%.

Calorie Know-How

■ Calories are the units used to measure the energy that fuels the body, generated when the carbohydrates ingested in our food 'burn' together with oxygen

■ The amount of exercise we do is directly proportional to the number of calories we burn

■ Weight loss is best effected by cutting back on calories consumed in food and stepping up physical activity

■ 600 excess calories a day can put on 1lb/450g fat

■ Even 100 excess calories a day over a sustained period will put on weight

■ Many manufacturers of food products now list the different food values as part of the packaging, a useful way to keep track of the calories. Get into the checking habit whenever you go shopping

■ The number of calories needed to maintain weight varies according to age, sex, metabolism and lifestyle (i.e. physically active/sedentary). As a rough guide, in order to lose weight a physically active person or one with over 2 stone/12 kg of weight to lose should cut down daily calorie intake of 1500; a less active person with less weight to lose could afford to cut down to 1,000 calories per day

■ A 10 stone/70 kg adult exercising for 15 minutes could expect calories used to work out as follows:

Walking slowly	55
Cycling slowly	65
Walking briskly	80
Dancing energetically	85
Playing tennis	120
Jogging	120
Cycling fast	168
Running	200
Playing squash	230
Swimming fast	255

■ The calorific value of different foods can vary widely. Here are 10 examples of high- and low-calorie foods:

High-cal (per 4 oz/100 g)		*Low-cal* (per 4 oz/100 g)	
Cashew nuts	610	Celery sticks	10
Milk chocolate	600	Fresh apricots	20
Double cream	510	Low-fat yogurt	75
Cheddar cheese	480	Cottage cheese	100
Roast breast of lamb	470	Chicken breast	160
Deep-fried scampi	450	Peeled prawns	120
Cheesecake	430	Canned sweetcorn	80
Pork pie	420	Plain boiled potato	100
French fries	330	Baked beans	80
Avocado pear	260	Tomatoes	16

Activity and lifestyle
The human body, which has been described as a perfect running machine, was designed to be active. Our early ancestors

were hunters, and relied on their ability to track their prey, for which speed and mobility were essential. To most of us today, a way of life that was once taken for granted would seem an impossibly tough physical endurance test. Our modern lifestyle all too often positively discourages physical activity, and our bodies quickly fall out of condition through disuse.

Muscle power

Over 400 skeletal muscles, made up of short fibres held together in bundles, shape and control our bodies, and play a crucial role in mobility and condition. The main function of the muscles is to move the joints to which they are attached smoothly and efficiently, sometimes with the help of tendons, by a process of contracting and stretching. Smaller, parallel fibres inside each muscle fibre slide past each other as the muscle moves, telescoping to make it contract.

Muscles tend to shorten if they are under-used. The more they are exercised, the more elastic, stretchy and flexible they become, putting less strain on the tendons, ligaments and joints, and resulting in a beautifully supple body.

It is not enough, however, for muscles just to be stretched: they need to be strengthened too. Through well-balanced exercise, muscles will also become that much stronger, providing the body with all the support it needs. Properly toned muscles make a much more effective natural girdle than any corset, responding quickly to energy demands and enabling the body to carry out strenuous tasks easily and efficiently.

Fit, conditioned muscles will also have greater stamina and endurance, will be able to keep up high levels of physical activity over ever-increasing periods and will consequently leave you feeling less tired, with more energy to spare.

Well-toned muscles have aesthetic as well as functional value. They look and feel resilient, and help to shape a body that will be tauter, trimmer, more shapely and firmer to the touch.

Fuelling the muscles

The energy to keep the body on the move comes from the muscles, which are constantly creating and expending energy. As in a car engine, where energy is liberated by the combustion of fuel and oxygen, so in the human body the muscles derive energy from fuel – most often sugars – derived from food, combined with a steady supply of oxygen. Food supplies the fuel for physical energy; oxygen is required for its release.

When the muscles are working hard during exercise, their oxygen requirements soar. A trained athlete may burn up as much as 5 litres of oxygen every minute – for which 150 litres of air are needed.

Oxygen is transferred to the muscles from the atmosphere through the bloodstream via the heart and lungs. The heart – itself of course a muscle – pumps blood enriched with oxygen picked up from the lungs, via the circulatory system of arteries, capillaries and veins. The blood supply varies according to the body's oxygen needs. When the body is at rest, the heart may need to pump only about 10 pints (5 litres) of blood per minute – but as much as 70 pints (35 litres) during vigorous exercise.

Exercising the heart

Exercise plays an essential part in your figure-firming plans, and a heart working efficiently to provide the muscles with the nourishment they need plays a key role in any exercise programme.

The extra demands made on the heart-pump by the exercising muscles for an increased volume of blood cause the dramatic rise in the heart rate which is normal during exercise. At rest, a normal heart beat will be about 72 contractions per minute. During strenuous exercise this may increase to 200 contractions or so per minute. Exercising regularly means that when the heart returns to its at-rest state after exercise, its rate will become lower, with fewer contractions per minute and lower demands made upon it. Body fitness, as reflected in body firmness, also means that the heart rate returns to normal more quickly after exercise has been taken. Top athletes may have a resting heart rate as low as 38 beats per minute, but a heart-rate of 45-50 contractions per minute would indicate a state of fitness to be proud of.

Exercising regularly improves the efficiency of the lungs and heart as well as of the other muscles. There is evidence to show that exercise increases the size and strength of the heart and the elasticity and capacity of the lungs, and also enlarges the arteries, which dilate as they distribute blood to the working muscles. If you are also following a low-fat diet, you are cutting down on cholesterol, the fatty plaque-like substance which develops in the lining layer of the arteries, causing the narrowing and blocking which leads to cardiac arrest. You will thus be taking a further important precaution to ensure a well-conditioned cardio-vascular system to support you through the most demanding figure-firming exercise programme.

Aerobic exercise

'Aerobic', which means 'with oxygen', describes any exercise which relies for its performance on an increased supply of oxygen. By making special demands on the heart and lungs, aerobic exercise works to summon up the extra oxygen the muscles need to cope.

'Aerobics' (see page 85) are just one type of exercise; others are walking, jogging, swimming and cycling, all of which are described in more detail in Chapter 3.

Of all types of exercise, aerobic exercise does most to condition the way the heart, lungs and bloodstream supply the muscles with the oxygen and other nutrients needed to produce the energy they are required to expend. In this way, aerobic exercise is especially important for the development of muscular stamina, although it contributes significantly to flexibility and general muscle toning as well.

Anaerobic exercise

Unlike aerobic exercise, which is essentially more prolonged, anaerobic exercise, which does not rely on extra oxygen, is done in short periods or spurts – usually under 90 seconds in duration. This more static form of exercise characteristically involves individual muscle groups, and while effective for increasing muscle strength, does little for enhanced cardiovascular efficiency. Weight-lifting is a typical form of anaerobic exercise; so are sprint or start-stop sports, and callisthenic exercises like sit-ups and push-ups.

Your personal exercise plan

When you are devising your own individualized exercise programme for firming your figure, as suggested in the next chapter, you should make sure that it includes plenty of aerobic exercise, especially sport, designed to condition your heart and lungs and increase your overall calorie expenditure, as well as exercises designed to target specific muscles.

EXERCISE VALUES

When you embark on a figure-firming programme in which exercise plays a major part, some of the health-enhancing benefits you may enjoy include:

- Strengthened and enlarged heart muscle, whose fitness and pumping facility improve as it is made to work harder

- Increased volume and capacity of lungs, boosting oxygen intake and facilitating breathing

- Dilated arteries, enabling more oxygen-enriched blood to reach the muscles more quickly

- Reduced blood pressure levels

- Increased metabolic rate, burning up more calories, after and as during exercise, and decreasing body fat

- Stretched and strengthened muscles, making for suppleness, stamina and good body support

- Enhanced skeletal tissue and bone mineral mass

- Increased energy and vitality

In addition, exercise may also help to:

- curb the appetite

- give up smoking

- control tension and stress

- create a sense of elation and well-being, by releasing the brain endorphins, the body's natural pain-killers

- create quicker reflexes

TWO

A Firm Commitment

Now that we've seen how crucial both a sensible diet and exercise routine are in any figure-firming programme, it's time to look at how you as an individual will work this vital combination into your life. Some changes, possibly quite drastic ones, involving some fundamental rethinking of the habits of a lifetime, may well be necessary. It's time to give how, when, what and how much you eat, and how, when and how little or how much you exercise, a fundamental appraisal, make the necessary adjustments and take the relevant action. You are basically going to be revising your whole approach to body maintenance, and giving it the care and prominence in your life which it deserves.

As regards diet, you will not be even considering following a 'crash' diet on which you may lose some weight fast, but will undoubtedly put it on again just as quickly. Nor will you be thinking in terms of 'depriving' yourself. Instead, you need to think in the long term, devising a healthy, balanced eating plan for yourself, which will suit your personal lifestyle and provide you with all the nutrients you need for energy to do full justice to your exercise plan.

Like your diet, the exercise programme you devise for yourself should be varied, balanced, interesting and enjoyable, and tailored to fit in with the kind of life you lead, both at work and at home.

Figure-firming is by definition a physical activity, but mental attitude plays an essential part in its success. It has to be something you really want to do. After reading Chapter 1 you know it makes sense, in terms of your health as well as of your appearance. But don't let this knowledge remain a general awareness; apply it to yourself and your body, and most importantly, start putting it into practice today!

Just as important as making the decision and taking the first step on the road to an enviably firm figure, is to remember from the beginning that this will be a long-term commitment – in fact, for 'long-term', ideally read 'life-long'. The right combination of diet and exercise can actually show results in as little as four weeks, and the first signs of success are tremendously satisfying. But getting into shape and staying that way isn't something that's going to happen overnight. It's a progressive, cumulative business, requiring effort, patience and above all motivation, so that your diet-and-exercise firming plan becomes quite literally second nature.

Your motivation has to come essentially from yourself, from knowing that you are doing something really worthwhile for yourself. Encouragement from family and friends can be tremendously helpful in maintaining enthusiasm and not becoming disheartened. Once you've embarked on your programme, there'll be nothing you want to hear less than that time-honoured, double-edged compliment, 'I like you as you are', so make sure the family understands what you are doing and why. Enlist their support and involve them too, choosing some forms of exercise in which you can all share, and making sure they too enjoy the benefits of your healthy eating plan.

You may also find it helpful – and fun – to share some of your exercise routines with friends, at home or in a class. And exchanging notes on diet progress with a like-minded friend, or joining a weight-watching group, can be a great way of maintaining enthusiasm and keeping yourself up to the mark. More of this in Chapter 8.

Remember, it's never too late to get your body into condition – diet and exercise can be initiated, and their benefits enjoyed, at any age. But, obviously, the earlier you can make the firm commitment, and stay with it, the happier you will be with your body – and consequently with yourself – and the easier you will make things for yourself later on in life.

So now you're committed and on your way, and it's Day 1 of your firming plan. This is when you need to give your body a close scrutiny, a thorough and absolutely frank assessment. Your findings will form the basis of the individual diet-and-exercise programme you devise as right for you.

A log book, in which you keep a note of your intake at each meal and time and type of exercise completed on a daily basis, provides a useful record by which to assess your achievements. It also acts as an invaluable aid to ensuring good overall balance and a spur to continued progress. An office diary, with plenty of room for daily notes in sufficient detail to be of real use, is ideal, and very well worth the few minutes each day that keeping it up-to-date involves.

Your very first entry in your new log book will be the results of your home-screening test. To carry out this test stand naked – or wearing only underclothes if you prefer – in front of a full-length mirror, adopting a relaxed position, i.e. as you normally stand in an everyday situation like waiting for the bus or queuing in the post office. Now check your posture, asking yourself the following:

■ Do your shoulders slump?

■ Is your back rounded?

- Is your neck at a sloping angle?

- Does your stomach stick out?

- Is your chest sunken?

- Is your weight unevenly distributed, with one leg taking more of the strain than the other?

If the answer to one or more of these questions is 'yes', then your posture leaves something to be desired. This is important, because good posture is absolutely fundamental to an attractive figure. However slim, firm and fit you train your body to become, you will never do it full justice if your deportment is poor.

Toning muscles will do a lot to help your natural bearing, and when your body is shapely and well-conditioned, you will have much more reason to want to show it off. But even at this early stage you can very easily show yourself how you *should* look. So:

- Throw your shoulders back

- Straighten your back

- Extend your neck, holding your head as high as you can

- Pull in your tummy and tuck in your tail

- Stand up straight with your weight evenly distributed on both feet

- Stretch up as tall as you can on tiptoe

- Breathe in deeply, and see for yourself how much better you look as well as feel.

Now, examine your body more closely, looking for specific areas which could benefit from some trimming, whittling and toning. Do you see any of the following?

- slack tummy
- sagging waistline
- bulging thighs
- drooping bottom
- flabby upper arms

These are the body areas where deposits of fat tend to build up most readily. In men, fat most often accumulates in the stomach area – the so-called 'beer belly' – and in women on the hips and thighs in particular. Make a note of the body areas which you think would most benefit in your case from special attention, so that you can match them up with the specific spot-exercises in Chapter 4.

Doing the pinch test

As mentioned in Chapter 1, fat should not represent more than 10-15% of total body weight, and it should be evenly distributed over the body, not concentrated in certain areas, as is often the case.

To check whether you are carrying excess body fat – at least half of our total body fat lies directly beneath the skin – try the pinch test in the following areas:

- Back of the upper arm between shoulder and elbow
- The back, just below the shoulder blade
- The waist

As you pinch, you should not be able to grasp more than a 1 inch (2.5 cm) skin fold between your finger and your thumb. If you can, then you need to lose some weight.

Body measurements

Taking accurate body measurements is a reliable method of assessing whether your body is in proportion, calculating your ideal number of inches to lose through slimming and firming, and monitoring your progress. How you feel in your clothes is also a good guide – blouses that no longer strain at the buttons, waistbands that don't cut into your midriff, and trousers that fit snugly and smoothly over the hips without the least sign of a wrinkle or a telltale pantie line are all very encouraging signs that the firming process is working! Not only will you look good but also feel good.

The body areas that benefit most from measuring are the bust, waist, hips, thighs and upper arms. Make a note of these in a measurement record chart, which you can usefully update every 10 days or so.

When you measure, make sure that all your muscles are relaxed, and don't cheat by pulling too hard on the tape measure – it should not be stretched taut!

As a general guide to well-balanced body proportions in women:

- Bust and hips should measure the same

- Waist should be 10 inches (25 cm) less than the bust

- Thighs should be 6 inches (15 cm) less than the waist

- Upper arms should be double the size of the wrists.

In men, the waist may be up to 5 inches (12.5 cm) less than the chest measurement.

Waist/hip ratio

You can use your body measurements to make a further body-fat test. Using a calculator, simply divide your waist measurement by your hip measurement. The highest healthy ratios that result are:

   0.8 for women
   1.0 for men

Thus, for example, if a woman's waist measures 29 inches (73.5 cm) and her hips 39 inches (99 cm), then her waist/hip ratio will be 0.74 – just inside the acceptable limit. But anything above will be an indication of excess body fat.

Weighing-in
Taking measurements as described above is the most reliable way of assessing where you need to lose weight and concentrate on body firming. However, you will undoubtedly also want to weigh yourself as part of your home-screening.

As mentioned in Chapter 1, charts expressing ideal weight in terms of height can be misleading as they do not distinguish between fat/muscle weight. If you do use such a chart, make sure that it distinguishes between body types, i.e. small, medium or large frame – this can make a considerable difference.

THE WRIST TEST

To find out whether your body belongs to the small/medium/large frame category, do an easy test by simply measuring the circumference of your wrist with a tape measure. According to the result, assess your frame type as follows:

        Small: less than 5½ inches (14 cm)
        Medium: 5½-6½ inches (14-16 cm)
        Large: over 6½ inches (16 cm)

When you weigh yourself, make sure that the result is as accurate as possible by using balance scales, which are much more precise than the spring type with a dial – these can vary quite widely in their readings. Ideally, weigh yourself in the nude or wearing only underclothes: if this is not possible, remove your shoes and outer garments – coat, jacket, cardigan or heavy jumper – first. Try to remember to wear the same clothes on subsequent weigh-ins, to give yourself a fair idea of your progress.

When you weigh yourself, make sure that your bladder is empty, and that you have not eaten recently. Try to weigh yourself at the same time of day – first thing in the morning is best. Women who suffer from fluid retention at the time of their periods should remember that this can make a difference of 2-3 lb (1-1.5 kg) to their weight.

Avoid the temptation of weighing yourself too often – this can be misleading. Weight does not come off steadily, but rather in fits and starts, and too frequent weighing can prove discouraging. Once a week is quite enough.

Finding time for exercise

Now that you have assessed yourself and made a note of your vital statistics, it's time to think about putting your exercise programme into practice.

It's a reflection on the age we live in that we should have to make time for something as fundamentally important as exercise, but finding the time can be a real problem for many people. For most of us today life is hectic, often a balancing act between handling a job and running a home, beset by pressures and stress created by both domestic and work commitments. One of the many positive benefits that exercise has to offer is that it can do so much to relieve this very tension –

in itself a good enough reason for making the effort to make the time. It's really a question of fixing a date with yourself that you know you will be able and will want to keep.

We have already seen in Chapter 1 how a combination of different types of exercise – aerobic and specifically spot-toning – is ideal in any figure-firming programme. For exercises you decide to do by yourself at home, set aside a time that fits into your daily schedule easily. For example, if you are out at work all day, exercising when you return home, before sitting down to an evening meal, may be especially re-laxing and invigorating – and better for you than instantly col-lapsing with a gin and tonic!

Some people find the idea of early morning exercise appealing, as a way of getting off to a good start, but it is not advisable to tax muscles that have not yet had a chance to warm up fully. You should not exercise for the first 20 minutes after rising, and over-strenuous exercise first thing may counteract the relaxing benefits of a good night's sleep. By the same token, exercising late at night may prove too stimulating and make it difficult for you to go to sleep easily.

Avoid exercising after soaking in a hot bath, when the mus-cles will be too relaxed to function at their best, or after a heavy meal, when making extra oxygen demands on the system will interfere with the digestive processes.

Whatever time of day you choose to exercise, remember that it is *regular* exercise that will firm your body. Sporadic, intermittent exercise will not have the same beneficial effect and may even be harmful if undertaken too energetically.

Joining a weekly exercise class at a set time on a set day is fun and a fine way of keeping yourself up to the mark on a regular basis. You can note the day and time in your diary and make sure that nothing else interferes with keeping the date.

But it's equally important to be as firm with keeping exercise dates at home: plan a convenient time slot in your day, and stay committed to it. Think of it as a treat, a special time that you set aside just for yourself. Make sure you get the very most out of it, switching off from the demands of the day and returning to your routine refreshed and invigorated.

Easy does it

Just as it needs to be done regularly, exercise should also be progressive. Once you've made your firm commitment, it can be tempting to let your enthusiasm run away with you, to rush into things, take on too much, set yourself targets that you cannot realistically keep, and incidentally increase the likelihood of strain or injury. You cannot firm muscles overnight – it's a gradual process that needs to be built up slowly.

So don't make yourself promises you will be unable to keep by planning lengthy exercise sessions and crowding your diary with dates. You'll run a very real risk of getting disheartened and this is when all too many people give up.

A realistic but attractively varied exercise programme could look like this:

- 3 exercise sessions of 20–30 minutes a day, including warm-ups and cool-downs, either at home or in a fitness studio
- 1 weekly keep-fit, dance, yoga or aerobics class
- 1 weekly swim or jogging session

Plus plenty of brisk walking or cycling in between.

Enjoying exercise

Devising a varied exercise programme not only works a maximum number of muscle groups, making for all-over body toning, but it also does a lot to counter the monotony factor which, like taking on too much to begin with, can so easily interfere with progress. Many people give up on exercise simply because they get bored with it. To avoid this happening to you, choose a number of different kinds of exercise all of which you genuinely enjoy – this way you'll be much less likely to fall by the wayside.

Exercise is a discipline but not a chore. Pleasurable exercise can become addictive!

Joining a health club

Some of the facilities offered by health clubs and fitness studios are covered in Chapters 5 and 6. Expert fitness assessments and supervision, a wide range of fitness equipment and other facilities, plus the pleasant social atmosphere of a club offering the chance to meet other like-minded people, make membership of a well-run health club an attractive proposition for anyone embarking on a firming programme.

Health clubs and fitness studios are ideal for anyone whose home does not offer the right exercise environment. If you live in a small conversion flat, for example, space may not be adequate to exercise properly, and pounding the floorboards will certainly not endear you to your neighbours.

If you decide to join a health club, do your research carefully. There are many clubs to choose from but a big variation in standards. Here are some points to look for:

■ How genuinely interested in your requirements are the staff?

■ What is the quality of the instruction and supervision?

■ What training have staff received?

■ Will you be given a full initial assessment?

■ Will this be followed up by regular supervision and progress checks?

■ What is the range of facilities?

■ Will you be given the opportunity of a guided tour
before you decide to join?

■ Does the club offer special membership arrangements,
for companies, for example?

■ How accessible is the club to your home or place of
work?

The range of facilities is particularly important. Membership of big clubs offering the use of a swimming pool, sauna,
bar and restaurant as well as a wide selection of equipment, is
bound to be expensive, but you may well feel it is worth pay-
ing the extra money and be sure of maintaining your interest.

Accessibility is very important, too. If you have to make a
long or awkward journey to get to your club, the chances are
that you will never make optimum use of what it has to offer.
Avoid the easily made mistake of joining a club to which you
have been invited by a friend, however attractive it seems
during your visit, if it is a long way from where you live. It is
much better to choose a club in your own area where you'll
have the added bonus of making new local friends.

Exercise and lifestyle

The type of exercise you decide to do needs to fit easily into
the kind of life you lead, so that it can become a natural part of
it. It is also desirable that some of the exercise you choose to
do should not only complement your lifestyle but offer a welcome contrast with some aspects of it.

For example, if you have a sedentary, desk-bound job, you

will benefit from more vigorous forms of exercise, such as running or rowing, whereas someone with a physically demanding job may find the relaxation of a yoga class or a leisurely swim more appealing.

If you live in a city, hiking in the country at weekends, with the added bonus of fresh air and changing scenery, has a lot to recommend it. Whereas if you live in the country, you have every opportunity to jog happily along lanes and quiet roads without breathing in the traffic fumes which can spoil this particular form of exercise in town.

If you're in a full-time job, you may find an exercise class, a game of tennis with a colleague, or a swim, works well for you, especially if you can keep your gear at work. Some large companies offer fitness facilities of their own to employees – in which case you have only to make the most of these.

If your life revolves around home and family, make sure that even with the constant demands these place on you, you contrive to keep some exercise time for yourself. If your children are small this can be particularly difficult – teaming up with a friend in the same situation, or joining a mother and toddler exercise group (see Chapter 7) are just two of the solutions.

Best of all is to involve all the family in shared exercise activity, so that everybody can benefit. It is a sad fact that far too many people give up sport and other forms of exercise they've taken regularly at school, through their teens and into their 20s, when they reach their early 30s. For this is just when the body's metabolism begins to slow down and overall muscular strength starts to diminish – in other words, just when exercise is needed more than ever. It is thought that this trend may be in some way associated with 'settling down' into family life. So make sure that when you start your own family, 'settling down' doesn't mean 'sitting down'. Get on the move together as a family, and give your children the best possible start by showing them what fun shared-exercise can be.

Seasonal exercise

Within your personal firming programme, try to develop a range of exercises that can be enjoyed throughout the year, both indoors and outdoors to accommodate our unpredictable weather. If you play tennis in the summer months, you must be prepared to get on court much less, if at all, from November to March. It might be a good idea to take up badminton as a winter alternative.

Nothing can beat swimming in unpolluted seawater, but swimming in an indoor pool, especially if there is one conveniently situated near where you live or work, is ideal year-round exercise.

Cycling, jogging and rowing can be done in all weathers, and although most people would be less inclined to do them in the pouring rain, all of them can be simulated mechanically in gym conditions, or by means of machines that can be used in the comfort of your own home.

Everyday exercise

You don't only have to take up specific sports and follow special exercise routines to tone your muscles and firm your body. As well as these, you'll find a surprising number of other ways as you go about your daily round.

Climbing the stairs, for example, is excellent aerobic exercise, involving the same degree of exertion as relaxed running – you can even simulate stair-climbing with a Stairmaster exercise machine. You will do a lot for your condition by making a habit of taking the stairs whenever possible, as an alternative to an escalator or lift. One minute spent climbing the stairs uses up 10 calories – and every little helps!

In the same way, make a conscious decision to walk more. Experts agree that a brisk 20-minute walk every day is first-class exercise (see page 39). Make a pact with yourself not to get the car out for short journeys, and get off the bus a stop earlier and walk the rest of the way.

Cycling is superb exercise for the upper body muscles as well as the legs (see page 50), and using a bike to get to work or nip down to the shops, as well as for recreation, makes very good sense.

And it's surprising how many ordinary everyday tasks like cleaning the car, housework and gardening involve exercising a variety of muscles. Making beds, polishing the floor or sweeping the stairs, mowing the lawn (the hard way!), digging or weeding the flowerbeds may all seem less of a chore when you realize just how much demand they make on the muscles, and the calories they burn up can help the firming process! Digging the garden, for example, uses up the same number of calories over a 30-minute stint as swimming for the same amount of time.

Finally, make optimum use of times like standing waiting at the bus stop or sitting watching TV to maintain the good posture essential to body-firming. It's all a question of thinking firm.

THREE

Firming Up the Aerobic Way

The aerobic sports are the ones that provide the most dynamic form of exercise, depending on extra supplies of oxygen for their performance and involving regular, rhythmical, sustained movement affecting the major muscle groups. The big plus of aerobic exercise, as seen in Chapter 1, is the way it strengthens and tones the heart and lungs, thereby facilitating the transportation of oxygen to the muscles all over the body. Muscles toned through aerobic exercise absorb oxygen more efficiently and also convert stored fats and sugars from the body's reserves into energy more readily. Through the increased oxygen demands it makes, aerobic exercise is beneficial to the circulation: blood pressure and cholesterol levels can fall, the arteries dilate, and well-toned muscle can make all the difference here, simply because the oxygen-enriched blood can be pumped through lean tissue more easily.

Aerobic exercise, by nature continuous, is particularly valuable for figure-firming because it can be carried on for much longer periods than 'stop-go' type sports such as squash. Squash is popular because it is exciting, fast, ultra-competitive and an all-weather game, being played indoors, but it makes extremely tough demands on the heart, and is really only suitable for the young and already very fit. Squash should definitely never be thought of as a *means* of getting fit, and should not be taken up in middle age and beyond.

Tennis is a safer option and altogether better alternative to squash, but its exercise value depends entirely on the standard of the players. If 'play is continuous', with long rallies between equally matched partners who have acquired a fair degree of skill, then it will obviously be much more beneficial to your muscle tone and figure than a game during which you may actually be in motion for only half the time spent on court. To get the most out of tennis, for both quality of play and exercise value, keep moving all the time between strokes. If you watch the professionals in action – Steffi Graaf, the West German champion, is a prime example – you will notice that they are constantly springing and bouncing off the balls of their feet, and are never still for a single moment.

SLOW- AND FAST-TWITCH FIBRES

The muscle fibres divide into 2 groups: *slow-twitch,* which require a steady supply of oxygen to function, and *fast-twitch,* which respond to stimulus and contract much more quickly than slow-twitch, and operate on stored energy rather than extra oxygen. Aerobic exercise works primarily on the slow-twitch fibres; and stop-go, short-stint exercise like sprinting and weight-lifting, on the fast-twitch fribres.

The big five

The most effective and popular all-round aerobic sports are:

- walking
- jogging
- swimming
- cycling
- rowing

Although these are suitable for most age groups, it is advisable to consult your doctor before taking up any new form of exercise seriously, and essential to do so if any of the following apply to you:

- a heart condition
- diabetes
- high blood pressure
- heavy smoking
- back trouble
- obesity
- pregnancy
- age over 65

Warming up and down

Both warming up and down are very important before and after taking exercise. Warming up stimulates the cardiovascular system: it gets the heart going, increases the circulation, and makes the increased blood-flow to the muscles gradual. This avoids the danger of pulls or strains which can occur when the muscles are overstressed. Warming the muscles gently increases their flexibility and loosens up the whole body ready for exercise.

Start all warm-ups by running on the spot for a minute or two, to speed up the heart rate – 100 beats per minute is ideal at this stage.

Now warm up the muscles all over your body progressively, starting with the lower legs and working methodically through the steps that follow.

1 Stand 3 feet (1 metre) away from a wall.
2 Keeping the feet flat on the floor, extend the arms and lean forward to touch the wall. Hold for 5 seconds.
3 Repeat 10 times.

Another excellent way of stretching the calf muscles is to:
1 Hold on to a table edge for support.
2 Bend your right leg at the knee and lunge backwards with your left leg, keeping it straight.
3 Holding the left leg in the straight position, *gradually and very gently* lower the heel of your left foot until it rests flat on the floor. Do not force your heel down. Hold to a count of 10.
4 Repeat with the other leg.
5 Do the exercise 5 times for each leg.

Here is an exercise for stretching the Achilles tendons which joggers will find specially useful:
1 Stand on a brick or thick book (a telephone directory is ideal) with your toes near the edge and your heels jutting out.
2 Supporting yourself by holding on to a table edge, gradually lower both heels until they are flat on the floor.
3 Slowly rise on to tiptoe, then repeat the exercise 10 times.

To loosen the lower back:
1 Lie flat on the floor, both legs out straight in front of you.
2 Clasp one knee with both hands and pull the knee as far into your chest as possible.
3 Repeat 10 times for each leg.

To warm up the muscles in the back, sides and shoulders:
1 Stand up straight, feet placed directly below the shoulders, with your hands clasped behind your head.

2 Rotate the trunk as far as possible to the right, then to the left, without moving the lower part of the body. Repeat 10 times in each direction.

3 Do the same exercise again, but this time with your hands placed on your hips rather than behind your head.

4 Stand with your hands on your hips and your feet shoulder-width apart. Slowly rotate your head clockwise in a full 360° circle. Do this 10 times, then rotate your head anti-clockwise in the same way. This is also a good exercise for preventing a double chin from forming!

Walking

Walking is so much second nature as a means of movement that its exercise value sometimes tends to be underestimated. In fact walking is excellent aerobic activity, its basic movement being repetitive and rhythmical and requiring extra oxygen. The oxygen is used to release energy from the chemical muscle fuels – carbohydrate, in the form of blood sugar, and fat from the body's reserves. The average adult walking on the level at 4 m.p.h. will use up about 300 calories per hour; a hill-walker can use up to 4,000 calories in the course of an 8-hour day.

Walking improves the muscles' ability to utilize more oxygen and generate more energy, enhancing their tone, strength and stamina. The mechanics of walking also affect a surprising range of muscles by:

- flexing the ankle, knee and hip joints

- stretching the thigh and calf muscles, hamstrings, and Achilles and other tendons

- working on back, abdomen, arm and shoulder muscles

Walking is strongly recommended as a basic component of any figure-firming programme. Building up to 3-4 hours' brisk walking a week, and always ensuring at least 20 minutes per day, will show marked results in a matter of weeks. You should aim to be taking 90-120 steps per minute at the start of a walking exercise programme, and work up to a maximum of 140-150 steps p.m.

ADVANTAGES OF WALKING

Walking has so many benefits and so much to offer:

- It can be enjoyed at any age

- Taking place in the open air, it is especially invigorating

- It is also immensely relaxing, keeping you in touch with your natural surroundings as well as keeping you fit

- Walking is uniquely flexible: the length, speed, location and terrain can all be varied at will

- The monotony factor which can threaten the pursuit of some other forms of exercise is non-existent in walking

- It is enjoyable both alone and in a group

- Walking is an ideal activity for all the family to share in

---

Walking gear

As with all forms of exercise, the right footwear is essential, to enable you to carry on in comfort for as long as possible, and thus derive maximum figure-firming potential from your chosen exercise activity. Heel stability is very important: this can be quite adequately provided by well-designed, well-cushioned, stout, waterproof shoes with a good tread on the sole to prevent slipping. Special walking boots provide valuable ankle support when walking on rough, uneven terrain, but can be heavy, and unless you are going to do a great deal of this type of walking, you may find lighter, midweight boots – rather like specially robust trainers – a better option.

Clothing should ideally be worn in layers so that you can strip off as required. The body generates a great deal of warmth while walking, and the lighter your clothes, the more you will enjoy it. You should always be prepared for bad weather by keeping a waterproof outer layer at the ready at all times. This is best carried in a back-pack, along with any other special equipment you need.

For day-long walks the back-pack does not need to be a heavy rucksack – a light day sack is ideal, and there is a wide range to choose from. Make sure the pack is big enough to carry extra clothing, maps, packed lunch, torch, compass, etc. Pockets are useful for smaller items, making them more readily accessible, and check that the straps are broad, well-padded and snap-fastening. The pack must of course be waterproof.

Walking routes
To get the most enjoyment out of your walking, plan a linear route, making use of the special detailed maps available from the Ordnance Survey, National Parks and Local Tourist Boards. Way-marked routes make walking simpler and safer, and there is a vast network of these to cover – often, like the Coastal Path, the Pennine Way and the Ridgeway, through some of the country's most spectacular scenery.

When you are out walking with the family, including small children, it is wise not to be too ambitious, and you should always ensure that children are kept involved and interested. Even quite young children can walk surprising distances if their interest is maintained – by playing 'I Spy'-type games, or following a nature trail, for example. Babies can be taken on walks in comfort thanks to baby slings and specially designed back supports. Family walking is an excellent way of getting children accustomed to the idea of aerobic exercise from the earliest age, which will stand them in such good stead all their lives.

Walking clubs

You may also like to develop your walking interest by joining a club. At national level, the Ramblers' Association is the best-known of these, and has local branches nationwide. The Ramblers do valuable work by keeping ancient footpaths and rights of way open, and thus contributing to the preservation of an important part of our rural heritage.

Walking techniques

Brisk walking usually describes walking at a speed of 3-4 m.p.h.

Power-striding is vigorous fast walking, at 4-6 m.p.h. The leg stride action is extended and propulsion is facilitated and movement accelerated by swinging the arms.

Race walking is walking very fast, just short of breaking into a jog, at speeds of 5-8 m.p.h., or even faster. Competitive race walking requires very high levels of aerobic fitness, and is an excellent way of toning the heart, lungs and circulation. It exercises muscle groups all over the body, rotating the hips and swivelling the pelvis, pumping the arms and working the legs extra hard. In race walking, the feet characteristically land directly one in front of the other, so that movement is much more streamlined than in ordinary walking. The race walker moves forward in a continuous straight line, rather than placing the feet to either side of a notional straight line, as happens in slower forms of walking.

Walking with weights: using hand-held weights while swinging the arms vigorously, wearing a weighted belt or carrying a weighted back-pack are all ways that can be used to enhance muscle-firming while walking.

Walking on the treadmill: the aerobic value of walking is confirmed by the fact that the treadmill is an extremely popular and widely used piece of fitness machinery. The treadmill means that you can walk for miles without going out of doors, and can build walking into any exercise programme carried out in a fitness studio.

Jogging

When done correctly, jogging is excellent all-over exercise. Through the gently persistent, steady demands it makes on the body, it is especially beneficial to the cardiovascular system, increasing the capacity of the heart, speeding up the blood-flow to the muscles, flushing wastes from the arteries so that they expand and function better, and reducing cholesterol levels. For these reasons, athletes and other sportsmen and sportswomen jog regularly to keep fit, and an estimated 2 million people in the UK alone jog on a regular basis. It is a very popular form of exercise for a number of reasons.

As with all exercise, you need to build up your jogging skills gradually and patiently. Always remember that with jogging it is time, not speed or distance, that counts. 'Little and often' should be your golden rule. Don't make the mistake of trying to cover too much ground too soon: 5 minutes out and 5

ADVANTAGES OF JOGGING

- Healthwise, jogging enhances the body system's ability to assimilate and make better use of oxygen

- It makes the joints more flexible through complete and constant movement of every body-part

- Limbs become more supple and more shapely

- Jogging is ideal exercise for fitting into all types of lifestyle, as it can be done any time and in all weathers

- Apart from investing in a pair of good-quality jogging shoes and renewing them as necessary, jogging does not require expensive equipment.

minutes back is ample to begin with, increasing the time to 7 ½ minutes out and back, then 10 minutes each way, until finally you build up to a 30-minute session, which you should practise at least 3 times a week.

As with other exercise, the secret is to make jogging part of your everyday routine. It is believed that jogging for 15-20 minutes a day over 18 months can *double* the elasticity and capacity of the arteries, and the results will be equally impressive in figure-firming terms.

It is perfectly possible to jog in a group – with friends or other members of the family, for instance – but as finding your own pace is so important, many people prefer to jog alone. If you do jog in company, remember that this is a form of exercise in which there should be absolutely no competitive element.

If you feel you may have quite a bit of weight to lose, it is advisable to shed some of this before embarking on a jogging programme, as carrying excess weight can put strain on tendons, ankles, knees and hips. Always jog on an empty stomach.

The jogging surface is important. Start out on grass – ideally short turf, which is delightfully springy – and always prefer jogging on tarmac rather than concrete. If you jog on an indoor circuit in a gym or fitness studio, the floor should be specially cushioned to avoid jarring. Out of doors, jog on level ground to begin with, keeping hills as an extra challenge for later.

As you jog, keep your body upright and relaxed, with your arms swinging through smoothly as when walking, and letting your feet fall in a straight line. Correct foot action in jogging is heel-to-toe. Never jog on the balls of the feet. Your foot should strike the ground nearly flat, but heel first: you then roll along the outside of the foot and drive off the toes.

Jogging gear
There is a wide range of jogging clothes – some with designer labels! – to choose from for all temperatures and weather conditions. Although a track suit can be useful for cold weather, it should be lightweight. Shorts and a T-shirt are ideal for the rest of the year. Whatever you wear to jog in, make sure there are no restrictive waistbands, and that garments are loose-fitting (but not flapping).

Wearing protective bands can help support the ankles at first, but good-quality jogging shoes are absolutely vital for stabilizing the feet and providing the right resilience. It would be a very false economy to buy anything short of the best, and you should bear in mind that shoes need to be renewed after about 50 hours' jogging time.

JOGGING SHOES

Before you buy, check that the shoes feature the following:

- flexibility

- adequate arch support through an inset arch cushion

- slightly elevated heels to relieve tendon strain

- cushioned rubber soles

- heel counters to stabilize and support the heels

- snug fit with plenty of toe space, allowing room for expansion as feet swell: ½ inch/1 cm between big toe and end of shoe is right

- nylon mesh uppers to provide ventilation

- variable-width lacing holes to accommodate wide/narrow feet and hold them comfortably in place

Swimming

For maximum enjoyment while figure-firming, swimming is hard to beat: in fact, it is often described as the perfect exercise. Swimming is supremely relaxing, for the water counteracts the effect of gravity, making the body weightless. The water facilitates movement but at the same time provides natural resistance through its density. This serves to strengthen the muscles by making them work that much harder, and thus contributes a lot to the figure-firming process. In fact, *fast* energetic swimming can burn up to three times as many calories as brisk walking.

Here are just some of the benefits of swimming as exercise:

ADVANTAGES OF SWIMMING

■ The force of gravity does not operate in the water, so there is no pressure on the joints, making swimming ideal exercise for people suffering from rheumatism or arthritis (see Chapter 7), or recovering from bone fractures

■ Because of the buoyancy of water, which makes the body weightless, swimming is good exercise for pregnant women and people who need to lose weight

■ Swimming exercises all the major muscles of the body, improving overall flexibility, muscular strength and aerobic capacity

■ Because the body is 'cushioned' by the water, risk of strain and injury is significantly less than in some other forms of exercise

■ Swimming is ideal for all age groups. Babies of 3-4 months who have had at least one polio immunization can be taken into the water by their mothers. It is never too late to learn to swim, either

■ Swimming need never be boring or monotonous. Style and strokes can be varied, and the facilities offered by some pools do a lot to maintain interest

The arms and shoulders, chest and abdomen muscles are extensively exercised in swimming, so it combines ideally with exercise like jogging, which works the legs hard, in a complete, well-balanced figure-firming programme.

Swimming in the sea – provided, of course, the water is unpolluted – is especially invigorating, but for most of us this is a treat which can be enjoyed only on holiday or days out in summer. Fortunately, swimming in a pool by no means need be regarded as second-best. Swimming is in such demand that many public and privately run pools now offer a wide range of excellent facilities.

Olympic length pools are 50 metres. Twenty-five metres is the standard length, and 30-40 lengths in a standard pool represents a good average swimming session for exercise purposes. A small pool would be less beneficial, as it involves so much more turning and interruptions to momentum. The ideal water temperature is 80°F (27°C).

Obviously, swimming is going to be much more effective and enjoyable in non-crowded conditions. Fitness studios with pools sometimes offer the ultimate facility of booking your own lane, which must be regarded as absolutely ideal for figure-firmers! But public pools offer a range of different opening times to cater for different groups of people – parents and under-5s, say, or over-50s, or women only. Obviously, family times like Sunday mornings are going to be specially crowded, so avoid these.

If you can, use a pool where there is a separate pool for teaching and use by children (these often feature water chutes and slides, which children love, and if used correctly under supervision in safe conditions, can do much to enourage their interest in the water and swimming). The main pool may be divided into slow, fast and medium lanes, which can be a big help when you are building up the number of lengths you do in each session. The lanes may be increased to as many as six for competitive use by swimming clubs: you may well want to join one of these in due course, as an extra spur to your swimming activity.

If you cannot swim, you will find that many pools offer lessons in groups (usually 8-10), and once you have mastered the basics, you can proceed to a more advanced standard. Individual tuition is usually more readily available at private pools. It cannot be stressed too strongly that it is possible to learn to swim at any age, and enjoy the benefits of this magnificent exercise. And once, of course, you have acquired the firm, shapely figure which results from regular swimming, you can reward yourself with a really stunning new swimsuit, as figure-revealing as you like, in the knowledge that you will be looking sensational!

Swimming strokes

Crawl (or freestyle) is ideal for a good swimming workout. The arm strokes provide much of the forward propulsion, with the legs kicking from the hip and thigh rather than calf and ankle, to keep the body stable and balanced. To maintain a steady rhythm as you swim, breathe in and out evenly, rolling your head to the side as you breathe air in, rather than interrupting the natural flow by lifting your head out of the water.

Breaststroke: a very good all-round stroke, gentler than the crawl, with more of a gliding action. It is perfectly possible to swim fast with the breaststroke, however: push as hard as you can against the water, circling the arms as wide as possible, and kicking hard with the legs from the hips.

Backstroke: a pleasant alternative to forward-propulsed swimming, which is excellent for firming the muscles in the upper arms, shoulders, back and midriff.

Butterfly: like the crawl, involves maximum energy expenditure, but in short bursts, so is less of an all-round stroke.

Swimming aids

Swimming normally, using any of the four main strokes, exercises all the body's muscle groups. However, if you want to concentrate on the *legs,* use a *kickboard,* holding it out in front of you to support the upper part of the body. To exercise the arms and shoulders by themselves, use a *pull-buoy,* two plastic cylinders joined by an adjustable rope, placed between the thighs, to keep your lower body afloat. *Hand paddles and free weights* increase resistance to the water and strengthen shoulder, chest and arm muscles.

20-MINUTE SWIMMING WORKOUT

1 Swim gently for 3 minutes, using your favourite stroke, as a loosener

2 Spend 5 minutes practising improving your strokes

3 Spend 10 minutes swimming 3 × 100 metres (or 12 lengths), resting for 1 minute after each 100 metres or 4 lengths. Ideally, choose a different stroke – e.g. breaststroke, crawl, backstroke or butterfly – for each 100 metres.

5 Finish with 2 minutes gentle swimming to cool down.

Cycling

Cycling is another superb form of cardiovascular exercise, considered by some experts to be as effective as running. It is splendid for all-over muscle toning and firming. As well as the strong, rhythmical, piston-like movement of the legs, the upper body is fully exercised as well, being used to balance and drive forward, while gripping the handlebars works on the arm and shoulder muscles.

Cycling is a delightfully versatile and flexible form of exercise. Cycling to work, to do the shopping, or even to pick up a child from school (providing you have a well-secured, custom-made child's seat fixed to your cycle), are all ways in which it can be made part of your daily routine, combining pleasurable exercise with convenience and economy. Although a good-quality bike – essential for safety and long-term efficiency – can be pricy, it is an investment that will pay handsome dividends, saving you money and doing your health and figure good simultaneously.

The faster you cycle, the greater the wind resistance and the better the exercise. Climbing hills involves working against gravity and so increases energy expenditure while helping you work more muscles than on the flat – for example, when you stand up on the pedals, out of the seat, to negotiate a steep slope. Multi-gear bikes – some feature as many as 25! – are of great assistance with hill cycling, but for most people a 10-12 gear bike will be more than adequate. The lighter the bike, the greater the achievement in exercise terms.

If you are considering taking up cycling as part of your figure-firming programme, go to a specialist bike shop for advice on the right frame size for your height. The positioning of the saddle and handlebars is very important too.

When you cycle, bend from the waist, keeping your back relatively straight; do not adopt a hunched position. Bend the elbows to help absorb road shock.

Pedalling in low gear at a high rate provides maximum exercise benefit. Change gear to keep your exertion level and cadence constant through changes in terrain and wind conditions. Aim to build up your cadence from 55-60 to 70-80 revs per minute. A tachometer fitted to your machine will gauge the revs automatically. Always change gear down *before* starting to negotiate a hill rather than when you are on it, to maintain a smooth cycling action.

Essential to good cycling is to know and observe at all times the rules of the road that apply to cyclists, as laid out in the Highway Code. Always be conscious of your road position, and never go out at night without lights. Wear protective headgear and bright clothing which is reflective in the dark. Avoid loose clothing that could get caught in wheel spokes and cause an accident, and wear cycling clips to secure trouser legs.

You can of course extend your cycling activity indoors by using a stationary exercise cycle (see page 75) which can facilitate a quite rapid loss of body fat, in conjunction with the right diet.

Rowing

Rowing is excellent aerobic and firming exercise, though it is not advisable to take it up after the age of 35, as it does impose extra strain on the back. Rowing is primarily powered by the back and leg muscles, especially the quadriceps at the front, and the hamstrings at the back of the thighs, with extensive use, too, of the arm, abdomen and buttock muscles. It therefore effects superb all-body muscle toning.

Fibre-glass hull rowing 'shells' fitted with a special sliding seat are infinitely lighter, more streamlined and better-balanced in the water than any rowing boat. They enable rowers to achieve much greater speeds at both recreational and racing levels.

Rowing clubs proliferate on rivers, lakes, canals and reservoirs. If you are lucky enough to live near such a stretch of water, you may be able to take up other water sports as well. For example, *canoeing,* which makes special demands on the upper body rather than the legs; *windsurfing,* which exerts the postural muscles ensuring balance; and *water skiing* which works especially on the legs and postural muscles.

Rowing machines (see page 76) closely simulate the movements and sensation of rowing, and by using one you can get an equally good aerobic workout without going anywhere near the water. But, of course, one of the great attractions of rowing is the very special view of your natural surroundings that it provides.

FOUR

Exercising at Home

Exercising at home to firm your figure has a number of advantages. First and foremost, it means that you can fit your exercise routine into your daily schedule more easily, finding a time that will not conflict with the demands made on your day by work, household tasks and social activities. As you will be exercising in the privacy and familiar environment of your own home, where you can play your own music and do your own thing, working out alone or inviting a friend to join you if you feel like company, you are likely to be more relaxed and consequently in the right mood for exercise. And if you are unhappy with your figure to start with – most people embark on a figure-firming programme for just this reason! – you need suffer none of the embarrassment which puts some people off joining an exercise class, particularly in the early stages.

That said, you need to be strong-minded to exercise successfully at home. Home surroundings can be distracting, as anyone who works at home knows, and plenty of strong-mindedness and self-discipline are required to switch off and not allow yourself to be side-tracked by domestic pre-occupations. Also, you will have no class teacher to encourage you.

The time

The time of day you choose to exercise is a matter of purely personal convenience, but do remember that your body is at its most relaxed and warm – as it should be for really effective exercising – in the evening. When you're feeling tired at the end of a busy day, the last thing you may initially feel like is exercise. But the tiredness, which is all too often the result of stress, will disappear miraculously after a period of controlled physical activity. Exercise is very good therapy! So do consider setting some time aside after you have come in from work, or put the children to bed, and use this time to exercise, as a natural transition from day to evening.

If you choose the end of the day to exercise, it would be a good idea to prepare the evening meal in advance – perhaps a casserole which could be heating up during the session, or serve a freezer to microwave dish – anything, in fact, that does not require your immediate attention.

Exercising first thing in the morning should be more of a warm-up routine than anything too intensive (see page 57), as your body has not yet warmed up sufficiently for the muscles to respond positively to the demands of vigorous, strenuous exercise. Taking a warm shower before exercising always helps in this respect.

During the day, never exercise directly after eating. Allow at least 2 hours to elapse after a meal.

If you have a baby or toddler, an obvious time for you to exercise would be during its morning nap. If you have friends or neighbours in the same situation, why not join forces to exercise, meeting in each other's houses and taking turns to mind the children?

Whatever time of day you opt for, you will need to set aside up to 30 minutes for each exercise session, and you should be thinking in terms of three or four such sessions per week, if you are to achieve the firm figure you are aiming for.

Having selected a time when you can be sure you will not be

interrupted, stick to it and do not allow anything to distract you. It's a good idea to take the telephone off the hook for the duration of the session!

The Place

The room in which you exercise should be warm in winter and cool in summer, and airy – good ventilation is very important. If you have a garden, exercising outside – on grass – in the summer months makes a stimulating variation to the routine.

Indoors, a full-length mirror can do a great deal to help your concentration and enable you to assess how you are doing; for this reason a bedroom is a natural choice.

Whichever room you choose to exercise in, make sure there is plenty of room for all the stretching, swinging, kicking, lunging and circling movements you will be doing. Move the furniture to make space and avoid knocking yourself.

Music with a firm, steady beat is a tremendous accompaniment to exercise, helping you to maintain and sustain effort and rhythm, and adding greatly to the fun of a workout. Cassettes and compact discs are a better option than records, as the needle can jump. Special exercise videos can be a great help too, bringing the atmosphere of a class led by a teacher into your own home. So make sure that your exercise room can accommodate a video.

Floor surface is important. If the room is not carpeted, an exercise mat will prevent slipping, as well as cushioning bones and joints, and protecting the back. You can buy special foam rubber mats from sports shops, or make an effective one yourself by sewing two old towels together.

As some standing exercises require support, make sure a table edge or chair is within easy reach. Some floor exercises involve wall support, so leave a blank wall space clear.

The clothes

Whatever you wear to exercise, it should be non-restricting and comfortable. Avoid long sleeves – a sleeveless vest or short-sleeved T-shirt is ideal, teamed with shorts or track suit trousers with an elasticated waistband.

Even if your exercising is strictly for your eyes only, looking as glamorous as possible will do wonders for your morale. A snazzy, slinky leotard with a pair of smart matching tights is a good investment for this reason, more than justifying the expense. If you enjoy wearing your exercise clothes, you will be that much more inclined to exercise regularly. Tights should always be footless, to prevent slipping. Leg warmers, like dancers wear, keep calf muscles and tendons warm and stretchy.

If you have long hair, tie it back in a pony-tail or keep it off your face with an elasticated hairband.

Do not wear jewellery while exercising. Dangling earrings, and jangling bracelets and neck-chains may look good, but they will interfere with your performance.

Early morning exercise

Stretching all of your body gently but thoroughly is an excellent way to start the day, and will get your muscles ready for any sports or more strenuous exercise you plan to do later.

1 Start by fanning out the fingers of both hands to stimulate the circulation.

2 Move on to the wrists, circling them outwards, then inwards.

3 Make gentle circling movements with your head, first clockwise, then anti-clockwise, to stretch the neck.

4 Shrug the shoulders up towards your ears, then roll them back in a circle.

5 Stand with your feet set about 18 inches (45 cm) apart, toes straight ahead. Stretch your arms as high above your head as possible, keeping your heels on the floor.

6 Swing your upstretched arms back and behind you, bending and flexing your knees as you do so, and without moving your feet. Dip down as deeply as you can, at the same time bringing both arms up behind as far as possible, and straightening your legs as you do so.

7 Again with your feet set 18 inches (45 cm) apart, stretch both arms above your head and, bending from the waist, lean over and touch your left toes with your right hand, keeping your left arm stretched out behind you. Straighten up and repeat, this time touching your right toes with your left hand.

8 Standing straight, swing the arms across the front of your body until your wrists are crossed. Open out both arms wide and swing them behind your body, as though doing the breaststroke.

9 Standing straight, right arm bent at the elbow, place your right hand on your right hip. Stretch your left arm out at right angles to your body. Gently bend the top part of your body over to the left, stretching until the side of your head rests on your left arm. Repeat in the opposite direction.

10 Standing straight, grasp one knee and hug it into your chest, keeping the other leg straight. Repeat with alternate legs.

Work up to 1 minute on each of the above exercises, repeating them as necessary, so that you build up a 10-minute routine.

Vary the toe-touching exercise (step 7) by sitting on the floor, back straight, legs out in front of you to form a wide V. Touch your left foot with your right hand and vice versa, keeping the other arm extended behind you. Return both arms to the upright position each time. Finally, make a double V with both arms and legs, by touching the toes of your left foot with your left hand, and right foot with your right hand simultaneously.

Exercise sequence

Doing a series of different exercises in sequence is far better than repeating isolated exercises. Your exercise routine will be that much more varied and interesting, and most importantly, will provide the all-body muscle toning which is essential to successful figure-firming.

If you find an exercise difficult to start with, the secret is to approach it gradually, never force it. This rule can be successfully applied to sit-ups, for example, which incidentally should never involve sitting up abruptly from a prone position. To avoid the danger of damage to the back, raise the torso to an angle of only 45° with the floor, rather than at right angles.

■ The simplest form of sit-up, ideal for beginners, is to raise your body 45° from flat on the floor, *keeping your arms by your sides*.

■ The intermediate sit-up is done with the *hands placed on the hips*.

■ Finally, progress to the advanced sit-up (most demanding on the abdomen muscles) by keeping your *hands clasped behind your head* during the exercise.

As you get into your exercise routine, step up its intensity and make it harder for yourself by doing more repetitions of each individual exercise, and decreasing the rest intervals you allow yourself between them. You can also create more body resistance by the use of light weights (see following chapter).

Choose a combination of exercises to work on different

muscles for suppleness and flexibility, strength and stamina. Ideally, you should start with the large muscles, in the lower part of the body, and work upwards.

To avoid danger of injury and develop well-proportioned and balanced muscles, you should also exercise both sides of opposing muscle groups, for example the quadriceps/hamstrings in the thighs; the external/internal obliques in the abdomen; and the biceps/triceps in the upper arms.

Spot-toning exercises

Spot-toning can make a very effective contribution to figure-firming, because it concentrates on individual muscle groups, isolating them and making them work extra hard. Remember, the only way to strengthen muscles is to work them-to the 'point of fatigue'.

Bottom firmers

Most of the largest muscles are situated in the lower body, so if they become slack through being under-used, the results will be that much more noticeable. This is especially so in the hip area, which is one of the places where fat deposits accumulate most readily, especially in women.

Anyone leading a sedentary lifestyle, at work or at home – or both – is likely to be that much more prone to a sagging, spreading behind which possibly more than any other feature can make an otherwise quite respectable figure look unattractively pear-shaped and out of proportion.

Here are two simple but effective bottom firming exercises, which work on the muscle underlying the buttocks:

1 Lie face down flat on the floor, with your arms by your sides and your toes pointed.

2 Gently raise both legs together as high as you can. Do not force this movement: you may be able to manage only a few inches at first.

3 Hold the position for a count of 5, then slowly lower the legs, keeping them straight and together.

1 Kneel on the floor, both hands flat on the floor, positioned directly beneath the shoulders.

2 Raise one leg off the ground, at a 45° angle, pointing the toes.

3 Continue to raise this leg as far behind as you can, keeping the hips square and without moving them.

4 Repeat the exercise with the other leg.

Bumping and bouncing, rocking and rolling on your bottom may not look very graceful or feel very dignified, but these are simple techniques which can work wonders on your rear.

1 Sit on the floor and roll sideways from buttock to buttock. To begin with, support yourself on the floor with alternate hands.

2 Progress to sitting on the floor with legs bent and the soles of the feet placed together. Clasp your ankles with your hands and rock from buttock to buttock, keeping your back straight.

3 Bounce up and down as hard as you can on your buttocks.

4 Extend the exercise by bumping yourself forward and back across the floor, supporting yourself with both hands, so that you are effectively 'walking' on your bottom.

The simplest way of all, but again very effective when done on a daily basis, to keep your bottom muscles toned, is to clench the buttocks, squeezing as hard as you can, whenever a suitable opportunity presents itself. Once you sit down and think about it there are numerous occasions – sitting working at a desk, or watching TV, are ideal moments.

Thigh-shapers

Flabby, bulging thighs are one of the most common figure faults, and also one of the most stubborn areas to get results from. For these reasons, most figure-conscious people pay special attention to their thighs.

Leg-raising is a simple but effective way to tone the quadriceps, the major muscle at the front and side of the thigh.

1 Sit up straight on the floor, with your back resting against a wall for support.

2 Bend your left leg at the knee and clasp it to the body with both hands.

3 Keeping your right leg straight, with the toes pointing upwards, raise the right leg first a few inches off the floor, then at an angle of 45°.

4 Repeat the same exercise, but this time lying flat on the floor, and raising the straight leg as far as you can in the air. Repeat both exercises with alternate legs.

To tone the inner thigh, where there is often loose excess flesh:

1 Lie flat on your back on the floor, with your arms extended by your sides.

2 Bend both legs at the knees, then lift them and open them wide into a V.

3 Fan the legs out to form the widest V possible, then slowly bring them together again. Hold both legs extended out in front of you in this position before re-forming the starting V and repeating.

4 The exercise may also be extended by crossing the legs after bringing them together, before returning to the V position.

Here is another quite powerful thigh exercise:
1 Sit on the floor, knees sharply bent and supporting yourself on your hands, which should rest on the floor as near to your body as possible.
2 Giving yourself support from your hands and arms, lift up your hips and move them forward in a smooth, gradual action, until your knees touch the floor. You will feel a quite pronounced pull on the front thigh muscle as you do this: never force the exercise.
3 Return to the starting position and repeat.

'Slapping' your thighs is done as follows:
1 Lie on your back on the floor, knees bent, feet flat on the floor, and arms stretched out horizontally on the floor at right angles to the body.
2 Keep your shoulders flat on the floor and hold your knees together firmly. Roll your legs over quickly to 'slap' the floor on your right, then reverse the action to 'slap' the floor on your left.

'Bicycling' in the air with your legs is also very good for your thighs, and as a general lower body toner:
1 Lie flat on the floor, arms by your sides, palms downwards, and hands tucked in below the base of the spine, to support it.
2 Bend both legs and work them alternately in a cycling motion, lifting them as high as you can.
3 Vary the exercise by leaning back on your elbows as you 'cycle'.
4 Make the cycling harder for your thighs by doing it with your hands clasped behind your head at the nape of the neck – you will feel the difference!

Tummy tauteners

Of all the body areas, the tummy probably causes most problems to figure-firmers, men and women alike. The muscles controlling the stomach are the least used by most people in the course of everyday physical activity, but they play a crucial role in the way the body functions, particularly in ensuring good posture and supporting the back.

The abdominal wall muscles distribute the effort involved in posture maintenance. The rectus abdominis, made up of two long muscles extending from the rib cage to the pubic bone, is instrumental in moving the spine as well as flattening the abdomen. Similarly, the external oblique muscles which keep the middle body supple, also play a vital role in flexing the spine.

So toning your muscles is going to help you avoid back problems, as well as giving you the taut, flat stomach which will do so much to enhance your appearance, whatever you are wearing. Don't be tempted to flatten your stomach artificially by wearing a control foundation garment. This will only constrict the muscles and weaken them further, and it is just these flabby, under-used muscles that put dangerous strain on the back.

Here is a simple tummy exercise you can do without even getting up out of your chair! It is a useful one to do at any time in the course of your day:

1 Sit on the edge of an upright chair, holding your tummy in and keeping your back straight. Hold on to the edge of the chair with both hands.

2 Raise your knees up towards your chest as far as you can.

3 Now extend your legs slowly and hold them out straight in front of you to the count of 5. Then lower your feet slowly to the floor.

For a floor exercise that works the tummy muscles, the curl is a better alternative to straight sit-ups, unless these involve the 45° angle as described on page 59. To do a tummy curler:
1 Lie flat on the floor on your back, knees bent sharply, feet on floor, arms straight out on floor behind your head.
2 Gradually raise the arms and upper body, bringing the arms over slowly in a fluid, easy movement to touch your toes.
3 Uncurl slowly and revert to the original position as 1. Then repeat.

Expand this curl exercise to work on the lower abdominal muscles:
1 Lie flat on your back on the floor, hands clasped behind your head at the nape of the neck.
2 Bend your legs at the knees, with your feet off the floor, and extend the lower part of the legs at right angles, so that they are parallel with your body.
3 Raise your shoulders gently so that they form an angle of 45° with the floor.
4 Extend your legs upwards, toes pointing out straight, until your legs are straight and your body forms a balanced V.
5 This exercise is made easier if you bring your elbows forward, parallel with your legs, when you clasp the nape of the neck as described in 1. It becomes considerably tougher if you do it with your elbows placed horizontally at right angles to your shoulders.

Another good exercise to get rid of 'spare tyre' is:
1 Sit on the floor with legs parted as wide as possible.
2 Lift your left arm above your head in a slightly curved position, and stretch and bend to touch your right foot with your right hand.

3 Return to the starting position and repeat on the opposite side. It is important to keep sitting still without moving your legs during this exercise.

Waist whittlers
An enviably slim waist, set off to advantage by a wide belt, is an essential part of every firm figure.

To whittle unwanted inches off your waist, firm it up as follows. First, with a simple toe-touching exercise, which could be made part of any stretching warm-up exercise routine:
1 Stand straight, feet together, arms raised high above head. Stretch up, pointing the fingertips upwards, as far as possible.
2 Keeping your legs straight, bend from the waist to touch your toes.
3 Return your arms to the position in step 1, then bend backwards from the waist, keeping your back straight.

'Turns' are also an excellent way of trimming the waistline.
1 Stand up straight, feet set apart, at shoulder level, with your right arm held extended straight in front of you at shoulder height, and your left arm extended horizontally, so that your arms form a right angle.
2 Keeping the hips square, and the legs still, turn the top part of your body only from the waist, first to the right, then to the left.
3 Do the same exercise with your right arm on your right hip, and your left arm extended horizontally, then in reverse.
4 Then do the exercise again with both hands on your hips.
5 Finally do it with your hands held behind your head.

Firming the upper body
In many people, the upper body tends to get exercised less

than the lower. Fortunately, the upper body muscles respond quickly to toning, and the use of weights (see Chapter 5) can be very effective in this area. These muscles are most adversely affected by the hunched posture, with rounded shoulders, which too many of us in desk-bound jobs adopt for many hours in the day.

THE UPPER BODY MUSCLES

Trapezius: shrugs shoulders and moves head
Deltoids: shape shoulders and move arms
Biceps: lifts forearm
Triceps: straightens arm
Pectoralis major: big chest muscle
Latissimus dorsi: big back muscle, with *teres major* and *rhomboid* in shoulders above, acting on the blades

---

Targeting these muscles through specific exercises can enhance your figure in a number of ways, including:

- attractively defined middle back, which looks good when wearing a swimsuit, halter-neck top or back-less dress

- firm upper arms, with no flab at the backs, so you'll look good in sleeveless tops and dresses, or T-shirts with short or 'cap' sleeves

- well-toned chest, which in women can give the breasts a firmer, higher contour

- altogether improved posture, with head held high, back straight, and shoulders drawn back

One of the best exercises you can do to strengthen and firm

the shoulder, arm and chest muscles is the *push-up,* which also works on the abdomen and back muscles as well – and your legs and bottom. The push-up is not an easy exercise, but is well worth persevering with, for the all-over toning it gives by means of resistance to body weight.

Start with a modified version of the push-up before proceeding to the classic one.
1 Lie flat on your stomach on the floor.
2 Cross your ankles behind you and raise them off the floor.
3 With your hands placed below the shoulders, elbows sticking out at right angles, raise yourself on your arms, keeping your torso straight, until your arms are straight and you reach a kneeling position.

Now the classic push-up:
1 Balance your weight between your hands and toes. Do this by aligning your body parallel with the floor, supporting yourself with straight arms, hands flat on the floor, and feet with flexed toes.
2 Keep your body straight in this raised position, supported by arms and feet. Do not allow your back or legs to bend as you lower your chest to the floor, bending your elbows.
3 Raise yourself again into the straight, aligned position, and repeat.
4 To use the push-up to work specifically on the chest, hold your elbows close to your body as you push.

Use the 15 suggested spot-toning exercises in this chapter as building blocks in your personal figure-firming exercise programme. Doing each of them repeatedly for 2 minutes would give you a 30-minute session – but don't forget to build in a few minutes at each end for warming up and down.

FIVE

Firming Aids

Now that you have acquired the exercise habit essential to figure-firming, and have got into a regular exercise routine, combining cardiovascular and all-over muscle toning with spot-toning exercises aimed at specific problem areas, you will be looking for new targets to set yourself and new ways in which to extend your exercising.

You need to do this in terms of increasing your body resistance, 'overloading' the muscles to make them work harder. An excellent way of achieving this is by using weights.

Weights You need special instructions in the use of weights, to avoid any possibility of strain and injury, either in the way you handle the weights, or in the heaviness of the weights you select. Weight-training has become very popular in recent years, and specialist instruction is now widely available in health clubs, gyms and local authority classes (see page 80).

Weights are of two types: free weights and fixed weights. *Free weights* are hand-held or can be strapped to the wrists or ankles to increase the workload. A *dumb-bell* is a short chrome bar with a set weight on both sides, easily gripped in the hand. Dumb-bells are useful for a variety of exercise, particularly for the shoulders, arms and chest muscles, when the basic pose is a standing one. As a general rule, women use 1.5-2.5 kg dumb-bells, and men 3.5-5 kg.

A *bar-bell,* or weight bar, is a long rod with weights fitted at both ends (these weights must always be equal), and is held in both hands. It is most often used to exercise the shoulders.

Strap-on ankle weights in a variety of sizes are especially good for exercising the legs and buttocks, and can be used when swimming. They are attached to the limbs by buckles or self-adhesive velcro strip.

Fixed-weight equipment includes single-station, variable-resistance exercise machines, such as thigh extension machine and leg press or hip abductor. In multi-gyms, a number of exercise stations are grouped together round a central block, making it easy to work steadily through them. In stack-weight equipment, the weights can be easily adjusted by changing the position of a pin in the stack.

Weights operated by a system of pulleys and springs in the multi-gym offer tremendous opportunities for figure-firming, increasing flexibility as well as strength, and effecting all-over body stimulation and streamlining. Elaborate and expensive equipment of this kind – well-known brand names are Nautilus, Cam Star, Eagle, David, Universal, Keiser and Tinturi – should be used in a well-equipped gym or health club, although some local authorities now offer them as part of their health and fitness facilities. But although free weights may seem less exciting in comparison with this hi-tech sophistication, it is very well worth mastering free-weight technique, because it can so easily be used at home, in combination with many of your usual exercises.

You should always start any weight-training programme at the lightest end of the range. Follow the advice of your instructor on when to progress to heavier weights. Perfecting exercise technique is more important than using heavier weights just for the sake of it.

WEIGHT-LIFTING WARM-UP

Take resting pulse rate.
Massage back of thighs, calves. Flex, extend and circle feet.
Stretch upper body (neck, shoulders, chest): 2 mins.

1 Bend head slowly to each side. Flex neck forward and back.
2 Stand straight, arms crossed in front at wrists. Swing arms out and above head, cross wrists again. In this position, stretch arms back. Bring shoulder blades together. Return to starting position and repeat.
3 Rotate elbows up in front, then circle them back and around.

Jog or cycle for 1 minute. Take pulse rate again, aiming for 25-30 per cent increase over resting rate.
Stretch trunk (back and abdominals): 2 mins.

4 Stand straight, legs apart. Stretch and bend gently to one side, reaching down as far as you can without straining, then hold. Repeat with other side.
5 Lie on floor on back; keeping lower back flat, raise head slightly, flex hips, stretch knees apart, bring together and repeat.
6 Still lying on your back, cycle with your legs.

Jog or cycle for 1 minute. Pulse rate should now be 50 per cent higher than at rest.
Stretch lower body (hips, legs, ankles): 3 mins.

7 Do wall-leaning stretch described on page 38.
8 Do double V stretch described on page 59.
Jog, skip or cycle for 1 minute. Pulse rate should now be 70-80 per cent higher than at rest.

Warming up thoroughly before working with weights is essential, to mobilize the joints and muscles and prepare them to undertake more strenuous activity, and to generate heat for more efficient body functioning.

Warm-up exercises could include circling of shoulders, arms and hips; waist turns; side bends; leg swings and lunges. Jogging and using an exercise cycle (see page 75) are good ways to warm up, too. See box for a suggested warm-up routine.

Skipping

Skipping is also good and is, in itself, an excellent cardio-vascular workout, which strengthens, trims and tones the legs and arms, and also improves balance and coordination. Weighted skip-ropes are especially effective for developing stamina and endurance. The right length is important: test this by standing in the middle of the rope – the handles should reach your armpits.

To skip, stand erect, elbows slightly bent, holding the rope hanging slackly behind your heels, which should be nearly touching. With a small, circular movement of the arms, swing the rope over your head and jump over it from foot to foot, as if running on the spot, springing from the ankle.

For warm-up purposes, aim at one jump per second. As skipping can be done anywhere, indoors or out, it would make a very good addition to your general firming pro-gramme, in which case increase jumps per sec to two or more.

Exercises using free weights

To tone the triceps and firm the back of the arms:
1 Lie on an exercise bench, on your back, holding a dumb-bell in each hand, arms fully extended straight above your head.

2 Keeping the upper arms still, slowly lower the weights several inches behind your head, so that the arms form a right angle at the elbow. Hold for several seconds, then repeat.

To exercise the biceps:
1 Stand up straight, holding a dumb-bell horizontally in each hand, elbows bent, so the weights are just above shoulder level.
2 Keeping your back straight, slowly raise your arms until they are fully extended vertically above your head. Hold, then repeat.

To exercise the pectoral muscles:
1 Lie on an exercise bench, on your back, holding a dumb-bell in each hand, arms extended horizontally at right angles to the body.
2 Bring up your arms gradually in an arching movement, until they meet above you and are fully extended vertically. Hold and repeat.

To exercise the leg, hip and buttock muscles:
1 Stand erect, feet set apart below the shoulders. Hold a bar-bell at both ends, elbows bent, so that it rests across the shoulders/upper back.
2 Bend your knees until you are in a half-squat position, with your thighs parallel to the ground.
3 Rise gradually until your legs are straight and you have returned to the starting position. Keep your back straight and your upper body still as you make the rise.

Exercise machines
The range of machines to help you exercise, including programme-planning and progress-assessment, is ever-

increasing. This is a big growth area in the health and fitness market, and an enormous amount of research has gone into perfecting highly sophisticated machines which are effective and safe to use. Users can set training programmes electronically to suit their own exercising requirements, and digital meters enable progress to be assessed continuously.

Exercise machines undoubtedly create incentive and impose discipline, as well as ensuring a thorough and efficient aerobic and toning workout. For all these reasons they can usefully be built into any figure-firming programme and become an integral part of it. However, using machines is best regarded as a means of varying the exercises you do regularly to firm your figure. Purely mechanical exercising would quickly become monotonous. But combined with the sports and other exercises already described it is of very real value.

That said, do think twice before investing in expensive machinery for use at home. Unless you are prepared to spend a lot of money on a top of the range model, and are sure that you have enough room to house it, you may well come to the conclusion that it makes better sense to make full use of a range of exercise machines in a well-equipped health club or fitness studio. Not only will there be a choice, but the equipment is likely to be of much better quality than home-use machines, and will of course be regularly serviced so that you are using it in peak running order.

Right at the top of the exercise machine range are the multi-gyms. They are effectively complete mechanical 'fitness centres' which can offer the facility to train muscles with more than 30 different exercises, such as sit-ups, lateral pulls, biceps curls, hip flexes, and a system of weights which can be selected according to individual requirements by means of an easy-to-use, precise and safe key-system.

Exercise cycles

These are probably the most popular of all the machines available. A sophisticated ergometer bike, designed to provide controlled exercise and measure fitness, might include the following features:

- adjustable saddle and handlebars to enable you to find the cycling position right for you

- sliding rather than fixed handlebars, enabling you to work the arms are well as the legs

- comfortable 'two-cheek' saddle

- weighted pedals with toe straps and variable load adjustment to increase resistance

- digital meter recording time/speed/distance/cadence and tempo (revs per minute)

- electronic calorie measurement table, showing you calories burned during exercise, with targeting facility

- pulsometer to measure and monitor your pulse rate

Exercise cycles fitted with a lectern between the handlebars which will hold a book or magazine will enable you to read as you cycle and thus cut down on the monotony levels.
Exercise cycling while watching TV is also a favourite combination!

Rowing machines

These provide excellent exercise for both the upper and lower body, being designed with a sliding seat to help you row in the ergonomically correct position, and simulate rowing closely. The load increases automatically with the speed, and digital meters display rowing time and speed, stroke count and energy consumption.

Treadmills

Basically motorized moving belts, these are especially effective for developing jogging and running skills, because resistance can be adjusted to create the kind of tougher conditions encountered when running up a slope rather than on the flat.

Other exercise devices for easy home use include:

Trim wheel

These used to stretch the muscles, especially the abdominals, by rolling a double-handled wheel forward and back from a kneeling position, following through with your whole body as you do so.

Thigh trimmer

This is an expandable strap attached to each ankle, providing extra resistance as you stand and kick to the side, back and front, or lie prone on your side and raise the upper leg. This device can also be attached to the wrists, to exercise and firm the bust line, upper arms, back and shoulders.

Finally, if you feel you'd like a break from quite so much physical activity, but wisely do not want to give up on the exercise which is the key to figure-firmness, you might consider taking some 'passive' exercise.

This is provided by the Slendertone machine, which exercises the muscles electronically, to give a concentrated workout to specific body areas. Plastic-covered wires connect to round rubber pads which are placed strategically on the parts of the body to be toned and firmed – usually the tummy, hips, buttocks, thighs and upper arms. The pads are held in place with elasticated bands.

Some people may find the sensation of the electric current activating the muscles rather strange at first. It is certainly curious to feel your muscles contract and work away while you lie prone without making any movement. Passive exercise can never be made a substitute for vigorous physical exercise, but can have its uses – as a morale-booster, for the inch-loss through muscle firming which the tape measure reveals can be quite remarkable, or if you have suffered illness or injury and cannot exercise as usual for a while.

Portable passive exercise machines are available for home use, but most people are likely to find a course of treatments on a salon model most satisfactory.

SIX

Exercising in Class

While exercising at home is particularly convenient because it can be done at any time to suit your general lifestyle and fit into the timetable of a particular day, joining a class has many advantages too. Here are 10 reasons why you might like to consider enrolling in a class:

Why join a class?

Regular classes help keep up morale and maintain motivation. A set time and place impose a discipline of their own, which makes a welcome change from self-starting exercise at home. However keen you are to do your figure good, there will always be times when you feel lazy, and at times like these there's nothing like a class to get you going!

■ A class gets you out and about and brings you in contact with new people, which can be particularly welcome if you are housebound for any reason. If you are at home with small children, many classes provide crèche facilities (more about these in Chapter 7).

■ In a class you meet like-minded people with the same aims, and probably the same weaknesses and problem areas too! Very few exercise classes are really like the pictures you see in fitness books, so even if you are deeply dissatisfied with your figure when you start, don't let this put you off joining a class. You're bound to meet people who feel the same – and probably look worse – and you are likely to pick up some useful figure-firming tips in after-class chat.

■ The common enthusiasm, energy and sheer body heat generated in a class are infectious and stimulating.

■ Although in a class you are all working together, rather than in isolation, an element of competition is often present too, and this can have very positive effects. Exercise is not of its nature competitive, but being aware of just how far the people around you are stretching, how deep they are bending, or just how high they are kicking their legs, can spur you on to do the same, or better.

■ There is such a wealth of different kinds of exercise you can learn in class – this chapter looks at just some of them – that there's no chance of getting bored.

■ Some forms of exercise – yoga, for example – must be learned in class with a qualified teacher, to avoid the danger of strain and injury.

■ You will be able to practise what you learn in class at home, consolidating and adding new exercises to your repertoire.

■ Most importantly, you will be led by a teacher, whose role is not only to explain and demonstrate, but also to encourage, inspire, and transmit enthusiasm. Your teacher will work along with you, modelling the exercises for you to follow, and moving about among the class, offering personal guidance, as well. Identifying with a good teacher can make all the difference to figure-firming progress in a class context. In fact the teacher is rather like a conductor with an orchestra, in relation to the members of the class, and his or her personality, initiative and imagination can make a very appreciable contribution to collective and individual success.

■ The best thing of all about class work is that it is such fun – and as with anything you do, if you're really enjoying exercising, you'll be that much more likely to work at it and keep it up.

Which class?

As mentioned above, you're spoilt for choice when it comes to deciding what type of exercise class to join! Fitness studios, health clubs and sport and leisure centres will usually gladly allow you to sit in on a class to give you an idea of what's involved before you register, and you may find it very helpful to do this. Everyone has special exercising preferences, and what's right for one type of body build, say, may not be for another.

Local authorities run extensive exercise programmes catering for all those wishing to improve their general physical condition. You can find out all about these by inquiring at your local adult education college, library, or sports and leisure centre. With the ever-growing interest in healthy exercise for all ages, special facilities for parents with their children, and for older people, often feature on these programmes (see Chapter 7). There are also classes aimed at encouraging unemployed people to spend the extra time on their hands by keeping fit and trim. Classes cater for all standards and aptitudes, combining fitness with fun.

To give you an idea of the sheer extent and variety of different ways in which you can keep your figure firm and trim at any age (and at a very low cost), here is a selection of some of the local authority classes you can join. (Obviously, every area's programme will be different.)

- Body conditioning, using light weights, to increase strength, stamina and flexibility

- Body stretch: fine-tuning muscles

- Fitness for men and women (joint class, especially suitable for couples who want to exercise together)

- Keen fitness class (for people who are already in good shape and want to meet tougher targets to remain so)

- Fitness for the over-40s

- Fitness for the over-50s

- Fitness for the over-60s

- Keep fit for women

- Keep fit in retirement

- Keep fit for parents with under-5s

- Family workshop for mums and toddlers

- Keep fit to music

- Weight training for women

- Multi-gym fitness and circuit training : pre-booked fitness assessment and induction class attendance essential

- Aerobics

- Yoga (for beginners, intermediate, advanced)

- Yoga in pregnancy

- Ante- and post-natal exercise
- Margaret Morris Movement (see page 84)
- Music and movement
- Exercise and relaxation with special breathing
- Posture into motion: different aspects of movement
- Jazzercise: mixture of dance and exercise
- Twist and shape.

One particularly impressive figure-firming course, organized by a local authority leisure centre, and appropriately called 'Move It', involves classes seven days a week – early mornings, lunchtimes and evenings – with an average of six classes a day. Classes forming part of a course do naturally have that extra edge – the work is evolving and progressing, with recaps and consolidation, all the time. The 'Move It' classes are as follows:

- Body conditioning: complete conditioning work-out for the whole body, concentrating especially on firming problem areas – the abdomen, hips and thighs

- Shape'n'stretch: to give tone and shape to the whole body

- Tone'n'stretch: working on isolated movements for toning specific areas of both upper and lower body, alternating with stretch

- Low-impact aerobics: all the movements done keeping one foot on the floor, with no stress on joints or back

- Aerobics: light intensity moves with optional use of

hand weights for increased intensity

■ Cardio-workout (not for beginners): dynamic hi-energy aerobics, combined with muscular strength and endurance work

■ American-style tap dance

■ Hatha yoga: emphasizing stretching, breathing and relaxation, to tone every part of the body as well as releasing physical and mental tension

Lotte Berk

If the idea of taking a private body conditioning class-course with close personal supervision appeals, then Lotte Berk's famous 45-minute classes might well be right for you. Lotte Berk believes that everyone can acquire and retain a youthful, shapely figure, if they make exercise a way of life, and exercise every day. Fit and elegant, she is herself a tremendous advertisement for her success (she was born in 1913).

Her unique exercise method, which is very strenuous and demanding, combines the techniques and positions of ballet (she spent 20 years of her remarkable career as a ballet dancer), yoga and orthopaedics, in which she became interested and proficient after suffering a spinal injury.

Lotte Berk reckons that it takes about a year, following her method – and of course the right diet – to get the body into peak condition. Her classes are tough and challenging: if this is the right approach for you, then you can be sure of results. There are three Lotte Berk Exercise Studios in London:

29 Manchester Street, W1. Tel: 071-935 8905

465 Fulham Road, SW6. Tel: 071-385 2477

72 The Grampians, Western Gate, W6. Tel: 071-603 9309

Margaret Morris movement

Another unique system of exercise, movement and dancing training, in total contrast with Lotte Berk's methods, but also founded by a dancer, and combining elements from dance, yoga and physiotherapy, in which the founder trained at St. Thomas's Hospital, London is the Margaret Morris Movement. Exercises are graded through a series of 10 standards, to develop muscular control and coordination, each one being performed to specially selected music. There is a strong emphasis on artistry and free-flowing movement, and free improvisation and movement composition are integrated throughout as a basis for creative movement and dance.

The Margaret Morris Movement continues to flourish (it was founded in the early years of this century), both in this country and internationally. More information and details of classes can be obtained from:

Margaret Morris Movement Headquarters
Suite 3/4
39 Hope Street
Glasgow G2 6AG
Scotland

Keep fit

Although keep fit nowadays tends to project a rather hearty, untrendy image, compared with the jazzy glamour of aerobics, it has an interesting history, and its techniques are authoritative, comprehensive and widely established.

The Keep Fit Association is a national body, with regional offices nationwide. It was founded by a physical education organizer, Norah Reed, in the 1930s, inspired by the gymnastics classes she had seen in Scandinavia and by fitness pioneer Rudolph Laban's analysis of movement.

The Keep Fit Association aims to encourage the understanding of the principles of movement, as well as exercise participation. Teachers specially trained in body mechanics and the use of music in exercise, as well as first aid, coach classes which still reflect the source of their founder's inspiration: the exercises are based on the movements of gymnastics – turns, stretches, bends, lunges, etc. – rather than of dance. Devices such as hoops, balls, clubs and skipping ropes are used as part of exercise performance and add to the interest of classes, which usually last about one hour. Even if exercise classes are not actually described as 'Keep Fit' they are often structured around the Association's teaching methods – a tribute to its enduring success. Further general information and details of area branches can be obtained from:

Keep Fit Association
16 Upper Woburn Place
London WC1H OQG
Tel. 071-387 4349

Aerobics

Although, as discussed earlier, any form of sustained exercise requiring extra oxygen is correctly described as 'aerobic', the word is most often colloquially used to describe the fast-paced, demanding, competitive and achievement-oriented style of exercise called 'aerobics'.

Aerobics became fashionable in the 1970s, and Jane Fonda did much to give them their fashionable image. Her *Workout* book really put aerobics on the map, with its special emphasis on pushing yourself to the limits of your endurance, in order to achieve the famous 'burn'. In fact the fast pace of this type of exercise can actually involve a quite high strain risk, and a form of 'low-impact' aerobics is now often preferred in classes, certainly recommended for beginners.

Aerobics are tremendously popular because they are exciting, racy and full of variety. They draw on jazz dance, ballet, gymnastics and yoga for the exercise techniques they teach, to strongly pulsing, rhythmical music: musical tempo is a vital part of the enjoyment of aerobics. Excellent for cardiovascular fitness, aerobics are also great for muscle-toning and body-shaping, working on all the muscle groups by means of bouncy, 'on the spot' exercises repeated many times.

While it is perfectly feasible to practise aerobics on your own, with TV programmes and tapes including both instructions and music to help you, a class is ideal, not only for the motivation, but because aerobics are best performed in a studio with a specially sprung hardwood floor. (If you are practising at home, do your aerobic exercises on a thick rubber mat.) As the basic movement of aerobics is a bouncing one, carried out on the balls of the feet, you will need special aerobic shoes (not jogging shoes or trainers).

The instructor is tremendously important in aerobics, calling out instructions, keeping up the tempo and checking on individuals' correct performance to avoid danger of strain or injury.

Here are some of the movements involved in a full aerobic workout: twisting; punching; squatting; jogging; marching; spot-running; bending; knee-lifting; kicking; jumping; stretching; lunging; swinging.

Dance classes
All the special forms of exercise for body-conditioning described so far in this chapter draw strongly on different dance forms, integrating them into method and technique in a

variety of ways. Figure-firming through dance exercise has been given special individual expression by Phyllis Greene Morgan, an American Martha Graham-trained dancer, in her Dancercise classes. These are led by specially trained teachers, all with various dance backgrounds, who encourage students verbally throughout. Emphasis is laid in these classes on dance sequences and linked movements rather than isolated repetition of exercises, and students are encouraged to present themselves like professional dancers in the way they move and make use of floor space. Dancercise is at:

The Barge Durban
Lion Wharf
Old Isleworth
Middlesex
Tel. 081-560 3300 or 568 1751

Dancing is of course an enormously enjoyable social activity. It is all about communication between people – which is why a class environment is really the only way to learn to dance.

Dancing can also be one of the most pleasurable ways of firming up your figure. Once you have mastered the movements, skills and techniques of whatever type of dance you have decided to learn, and have been shown how your body should respond and adapt, you will have all the enjoyment of expressing yourself in a new dance-language, with infinite scope for doing this.

Dancing provides a terrific workout for muscular strength, suppleness and stamina – in fact it is a complete fitness programme in itself, using every set of muscles, tapering limbs, and improving the circulation and performance of the heart and lungs.

There is a tremendous range of dance forms to choose from: all are beneficial for figure-firming; all have something special and individual to offer.

Ballet is based on a rigorous, highly disciplined and precise training, with correct stance, body placement and positions of supreme importance. Barre-work is essential in the strengthening exercises performed in ballet practice, providing resistance as well as support.

Jazz dance, born in Black American culture, is highly versatile and exciting, with lots of scope for improvisation and creative self-expression, and for devising new rhythm sequences. It is vibrant, vital and sensuous.

Tap dancing, which originated in clog-dancing and jigs, evolved as a form of jazz dance. It is a wonderful limb-loosener, full of humour and fun, and based on steps that can be shuffling, or slick and snappy, and when performed by expert dancers, can involve thrilling displays of acrobatics.

Gentler, less strenuous dance forms are no less effective as a form of conditioning. Ballroom dancing, for example, though it often has special appeal for older people (see Chapter 7), is excellent for muscle toning at any age. There is also, of course, a colourful and exciting range of dance from different nations and ethnic groups.

Here are just some of the dance classes you will find featuring as part of a local authority programme:

- Afro-Caribbean dance
- Oriental dancing
- Ballet
- Ballroom and Latin American
- Old time and ballroom

- Contemporary dance
- Disco dancing
- Jazz dance
- Square dancing
- Flamenco dancing
- Tap dancing
- Scottish country dancing and national folk dancing of many countries.

Contact addresses
The London Contemporary Dance School
The Place, 17 Dukes Road
London WC1
Tel. 071-387 0152
(For information on contemporary dance.)

The British Council of Ballroom Dancing
87 Parkhurst Road
Holloway
London N7 0LP
Tel. 071-609 1386
(Publish a Directory of Ballroom Dancing Schools in Great Britain.)

English Folk Dance and Song Society
Cecil Sharpe House
2 Regents Park Road
London NW1 7AY
Tel. 071-485 2206

Society for International Folk Dancing
16 Bathurst Avenue
London SW19 3AE
Tel. 081-543 1891

Yoga

We have seen how dance steps, patterns and rhythms are incorporated into many forms of exercise, and the same is true of the movement awareness techniques of yoga.

The Eastern philosophy of yoga, which originated in India some 5,000 years ago, emphasizes the partnership of mental and physical discipline to achieve total fulfilment and control.

The type of yoga most commonly practised in the West is Hatha Yoga, which means the physical practice of yoga. This is the form of yoga taught in classes here, in which students learn the importance of concentration and body awareness, getting to know their bodies by means of slow, quiet, sustained movements and special breathing techniques.

In yoga, body fitness is acquired by the regular practice of a series of precisely defined postures or *asanas*, intended to focus on specific limbs, joints and muscle groups, and to massage the internal organs of the body, improving the circulation and assisting the digestion. *Pranayama (prana* means 'life force') are controlled breathing exercises designed to improve lung capacity and the respiratory system, and enhance concentration and awareness.

There are hundreds of *asanas*, some of them very difficult, which can take years to learn. In most classes in this country only a relatively small proportion of these are taught, in a combination of standing, sitting and prone poses. The *asanas* were originally based on animals' stretching movements, and the physical essence of yoga is to stretch the muscles slowly and gently without strain, relaxing into postures which are then held for as long as possible. The duration of the hold becomes longer with experience and practice. The *asanas* develop balance and poise, superb muscular toning and control, flexibility and suppleness. They also focus and absorb the practitioner's mental energies, resulting in the quiet, refreshed and revitalized mind, the state of total relaxation and inner peace which are the essence of yoga.

Training to qualify as a yoga teacher involves a rigorous three-year course, covering anatomy and body mechanisms as well as the philosophy and practice of yoga. Different schools of yoga all over the country offer different approaches to its practice, although the basic *asanas* and *pranayamas* remain the same. Further information is available from:

Yoga for Health Foundation (an international organization and registered charity)
Ickwell Bury
near Biggleswade
Beds
Tel. 076 727 271

The British Wheel of Yoga
80 Lecklehampton Road
Cheltenham
Glos
Tel. 0242 24889

In yoga there are hundreds of *asanas*. These are just some of the ones you are likely to learn in a yoga class: Locust; Sun Salutation; Cobra; Catstretch; Triangle; Plough; Shooting Bow; Staff.

SEVEN

Firm for Life

One of the most encouraging things to be said about figure-firming is that it can be successfully undertaken at any age. It's never too late to get into shape, and some aspects of the 'ageing' process, which perhaps we take too readily for granted, can be countered, if not reversed, by taking the right exercise and following the right diet to ensure a firm figure later in life.

However, this all comes much more easily if instead of having to break bad habits, you have from the start made figure-firming part of your everyday approach to life. If this is the case, you will be *maintaining* a good figure and well-conditioned body, which is a lot simpler than having to acquire a totally new shape. We all experience moments when it is tempting to 'let oneself go', and there are periods in life when for a variety of reasons we become particularly prone to such a tendency – many people find that this occurs especially in the middle years. But being aware, anticipating, and taking relevant action as necessary, means that figure 'afflictions', like middle-aged spread, by no means have to be taken for granted as one of the facts of life.

Laying the foundations

Body awareness is something from which we can all benefit, and from the earliest age. Parents owe it to their children to help them realize the value of taking exercise and eating the right kinds of food (for details of these, see Chapter 8), as part of growing up. The best way this can be done is by example. If you grow up in a home where physical activity is valued, encouraged and shared, and thought of as the greatest fun, and where a nutritious, balanced diet is followed and enjoyed as a matter of course, you really are getting the very best start in life as far as maintaining a healthy, fit and well-conditioned body is concerned.

A glance at any children's playground in full cry, with its scene of seemingly perpetual motion, is a very good indicator of how physical activity is normally second nature in childhood. Children usually require no encouragement to take all the exercise they need – just the opportunity, for them to be up and away. It is variety of opportunity and facilities, as well as interest and enthusiasm, that parents and school can most usefully provide, helping children to build up skills which if properly maintained will keep them in good shape for life.

These skills can be acquired as early as babyhood. Some local authorities feature endearingly named 'baby bounce' classes as part of their health and fitness programmes. Personally supervised by the parents, these aim to develop strength, balance and coordination in small babies, as well as providing endless fun on the trampoline and 'bouncy castle'.

As children get older, the whole family can benefit from family nights and family workshops, where parents exercise together with their children. Some local authorities organize after-school sporting activity sessions for juniors, as well as Saturday morning facilities and holiday classes. These are designed to encourage the children to try out as many different physical activities as possible, rather than specializing, thus laying a sporting foundation on which they will be able to build throughout their lives. This is a wonderful opportunity for them to find out for themselves which sports they are naturally best at and consequently enjoy most – and genuinely enjoying exercise, as we have seen, is the best guarantee of taking it regularly and thereby deriving maximum benefit.

Swimming is an ideal activity to share as a family, and this is encouraged by local authorities in special parent-and-baby classes. Here parents take babies up to the age of 18 months, and toddlers up to 3 years, into the pool, teaching them water confidence and the basic skills they need to learn to swim, under the supervision of a fully qualified teacher.

Once the children are old enough to take to the water on their own, they can join a variety of classes for different standards and age groups. Initially they learn the basic stroke techniques, progressing to distance swimming, and perhaps acquiring skills like diving, sub aqua and life-saving as well.

The Amateur Swimming Association organizes Swim Fit, Water Skills and Rainbow Awards, specially for school children, and these are a great way of stimulating and maintaining an interest in swimming through childhood and beyond. Information on these awards can be obtained from:

Miss L.V. Cook
12 Kings Avenue
Woodford Green
Essex
Tel. 081-504 9361

Parents of keen swimmers may also find the following address useful:
English School Swimming Association
3 Maybank Grove
Liverpool L17 6DW
Tel. 051 427 3707

Other leisure activities which lend themselves well to full family participation are cycling and walking, both of which can feature in an active and thoroughly enjoyable family holiday as well as in an everyday activity programme at home throughout the year. There are few better ways to equip children to enjoy a physically active lifestyle when they grow up than by encouraging them to cycle and walk – particularly if they are not particularly sporty. In fact, if children are not good at games in school, it's all the more important to interest them in becoming physically active in other ways during their leisure time. Above all, beware of your child joining the increasing ranks of children suffering from early obesity – these statistics are worrying, and the wrong foods, as well as too little physical exercise, must be responsible.

Children who show sporting aptitude are most likely to develop their competitive instinct as they grow into their teens, and it is during the teenage years and the 20s that most people are most physically active in their chosen sport. A tendency to lose this competitive edge in the 30s means that too many of us can give up sport just when we need it most – when approaching mid-life. So the message is simple – start early and maintain a lifelong interest in physical activity of some kind.

Teenagers who do not switch on to ball-games and are going through a stage when joining in team games is the last thing they feel inclined to do may enjoy an activity such as hill-walking or orienteering more. And parents whose children seem temporarily disinclined to take any physical exercise – or, it may seem at times, to exist at all! – away from the disco, may derive some comfort from knowing that disco dancing is one of the most energetic and aerobically beneficial of all forms of exercise!

Firming your figure after a baby

Getting back into good shape after the birth of a baby is absolutely essential for morale as well as health and looks, and also to provide the extra muscular strength you will need to lift and carry the baby.

Taking some form of gentle controlled exercise *during* pregnancy – swimming is specially recommended as exercise for mums-to-be – will help your body resume its former shape more quickly and easily after the birth. But you will inevitably have lost muscle condition as a direct result of carrying a baby, and you should aim to restore this as soon as possible. Talk to your doctor and health visitor about how soon after the birth they feel you would benefit from exercise. It may be advisable to leave embarking on a full routine until after your first post-natal (six-week) visit, or you may be able to start some not too strenuous exercising sooner.

During pregnancy the muscles of the abdomen, pelvic floor and rib-cage have been extensively stretched, and will feel slack and weak after the event. Other muscles, too, will have lost tone, as a result of restricted physical activity during the latter stages of pregnancy – another good reason for making a habit of exercising before your baby is born. Ligaments, especially of the spine and pelvis, will have softened and stretched due to the influence of the progesterone and relaxin hormones, and you will want to pay special attention to strengthening your back.

Your breasts will have enlarged substantially during pregnancy, and if you are breast-feeding especially, may tend to droop and sag. A special supporting maternity bra wil help in the short term, but chest-toning exercises, which work on the pectoral muscles supporting the breasts, will be highly beneficial.

Your overall posture may have suffered while you have been carrying the baby, with the gradual increase and changed distribution of weight. You may find your shoulders have grown rounded and your spine hollowed, and that you have adopted a backward-leaning stance. Now is the time to correct all these points, by making a fresh reassessment of your posture, as described in Chapter 2.

The bottom-firming, tummy-tautening and waist-whittling spot-toning exercises given in Chapter 4 will work well during the post-natal period. Here are some further exercise suggestions which will be particularly effective:

Arching your back like a cat will strengthen your abdominal and buttock muscles as well as doing your back good:
1 Kneel on the floor on all fours.
2 Breathing out, arch your back and tuck in your abdomen and buttocks so that your pubic bone moves forward.
3 Hold to the count of 4, then gently relax until your back is flat again.

The hammock of muscles below the pelvis, known as the pelvic floor, get enormously stretched during pregnancy, for it is these muscles, surrounding the urethra, vagina and anus, that carry the full weight of the baby in the uterus. Learning to contract the pelvic floor muscles – which can be quite hard work at first – will not just help your shape and posture, but will enhance your sex life as well.
1 Lie on a bed or cushioned on the floor.
2 Tighten the ring of muscles around your anus, hold, then relax.
3 Draw your vaginal muscles in and up as though gripping a tampon. Hold the muscles braced to a count of 4, then relax.

When you feel ready to, make your pelvic floor muscles work harder by repeating these exercises in a squatting position.
Here are three simple but effective exercises to tone your bust:

1 Stand up straight, elbows bent, fingertips touching at chin level.
2 Keeping the arms at shoulder level, but releasing the fingertips, pull the elbows back as far as possible behind the shoulders.
3 Return to the starting position and repeat.

1 Sit straight on a chair, feet and knees apart.
2 Lift your arms and bend them in front of you at the elbows, so that you are holding each upper arm with the opposite hand.
3 Push your palms firmly against your upper arms, feeling your pectoral muscles contract as you do so. Stop pushing and feel the muscles relax.

1 Stand erect, resting the fingertips of each hand on either shoulder.
2 Still touching your shoulders in this position, bring your elbows back and draw circles with them in a backwards, then forwards movement. Make the circles as large and complete as you can.

While exercising at home after giving birth can be conveniently fitted around those times during the day when the baby is asleep, it does require special discipline on the part of a new mother, who suddenly finds herself with a lot to cope with. For this reason, many women in this situation find special post-natal exercise classes with crèche facilities invaluable. Investigate the possibilities available through your local adult education institute, or get informed through the National Childbirth Trust, who do excellent work in this respect, organizing classes through local groups on a nationwide basis:

The National Childbirth Trust
Alexandra House
Oldham Terrace
London W3 6NH
Tel. 081-992 6762

Mid-life

As we get older, our muscular strength tends to decline and our metabolism to slow down. Far from justifying settling back into a less active lifestyle, however, these changes should act as a very real incentive to maintain regular exercise. Muscles that are regularly toned and persistently exercised will remain supple and elastic for longer, making movements of the joints and limbs easier. Exercise will also keep the body's metabolism stimulated, and the energy equation (see page 11) in balance.

For too many women, however, the menopause, which usually occurs in the late 40s and early 50s, means the loss of what may have previously been a fine figure. Yet the belief that this is inevitable is just another of the myths that still surround this period in a woman's life.

In physical terms, the menopause is a time of hormonal change, with a particularly marked falling-off in the level of oestrogen-secretion in the body. The pelvic floor muscles tend to become flabby and to lose their elasticity, and there is some redistribution of body fat from the arms and legs to the shoulders, buttocks and abdomen, which makes a general tendency to gain weight at this time more noticeable.

The mood changes and fits of depression commonly (though by no means always) associated with the duration of the menopause may be exacerbated in the woman by the experience of a slackening body. A waist that is allowed to thicken and an outline allowed to lose its former trimness may only confirm in some women what they are already feeling – that they are losing their sexual attraction. These negative, usually unfounded, feelings may also coincide with a time in a woman's life when she suddenly finds herself experiencing unfamiliar feelings of worthlessness, now that her children have grown up and she has much less to do than formerly.

This is much too precious a time to let yourself sink into a state of inactivity or even lethargy. On the contrary, now is the moment in your life to develop and pursue interests for which there was too little time before. Now, too, is the time to boost your own self-esteem and project a positive image by making sure you look as good, if not better, than ever before figure-wise, watching your diet (see Chapter 8), developing a home exercise programme, and joining one of the many classes open to you.

Cellulite

In middle age, particularly, women are often afflicted by unattractive lumpy, rather suet-like fatty tissue which accumulates in the hip, thigh and upper arm areas. The tell-tale signs of the condition known as cellulite are a dimpled, 'orange-peel' effect on the skin surface, and the longer it is allowed to accumulate, the harder and more engrained it becomes.

Cellulite, which is an exclusively feminine condition, is also something of a controversial issue. It has been taken seriously in France for a number of years but in this country opinion differs considerably as to its cause. One theory is that it is initially caused by the stagnation of blood in the capillaries, and exacerbated by poor circulation – often as the result of a too sedentary lifestyle with insufficient exercise, which makes it difficult for the lymph nodes to drain away excess fluid. When this is retained, the cells become waterlogged and loaded with toxins – hence the characteristically 'spongy' texture of cellulite.

Coping with cellulite

Dispersing cellulite will do wonders to help you achieve a sleek, firm outline. Here are some suggestions for getting to grips with it:

- Avoid junk foods and fats, and too much salt, sugar, caffeine and alcohol in the diet.

- Eat plenty of raw foods, especially fresh fruit and vegetables.

- Other sources of fibre, grains and pulses, for instance, can be particularly valuable additions to the diet as some experts believe sluggish bowels contribute to cellulite.

- Lymphatic drainage massage, a hard, tough form of massage, which dilates the blood vessels to improve the circulation, works on the principle that cellulite is formed as described above. The application of pressure to the body's lymph points with pummelling and kneading activates the lymph nodes and helps to disperse the cellulite deposits.

- Aromatherapy massage oils in which a sweet almond or jojoba oil base is blended with pure essential oils – highly concentrated essences extracted from flowers and herbs –

are readily absorbed through the skin and taken into the bloodstream. A specially developed cellulite oil contains lavender, cypress and juniper (a diuretic), to tone up the circulation and stimulate the lymphatic drainage system, encouraging the body to disperse and excete the retained fluid and toxins which are the root cause of cellulite. After massaging the cellulite areas with a loofah or special hand mitt in a warm bath, the oil is applied in an upward stroking movement.

■ G-5 massage. This electrically operated massage machine is specially designed to work on cellulite areas. The deep-vibratory massage breaks down fatty deposits, tones up the circulation, and flushes out wastes and toxins through the lymphatic drainage system. A course of a minimum of five treatments is usually recommended.

Retirement

This period in life, now frequently referred to as the 'Third Age' is starting earlier and earlier for many people – often in the 50s rather than the 60s.

Whenever retirement comes for you, it is something to look forward to, plan for and treasure. Your time is your own at last, and it is up to you to make the best use of it.

Keeping fit plays an essential part in retirement. In fact you can look forward to becoming even fitter after you retire than before, with more time available and greater flexibility as to how you spend your day.

Although retirement brings a well-earned respite from the pressures and strictures of working life, it is emphatically not a time for putting your feet up and taking life too easy in a physical sense. In fact it is now thought that some of the 'normal symptoms' of ageing, such as changes in the cardiovascular and respiratory system, cholesterol levels, bone mineral mass and joint flexibility, may be the result of inactivity rather than the inevitable process of getting older.

Exercising regularly will help you maintain strength in muscles which tend to shorten with age; keep your body from slackening and looking old; and ensure that your mental reactions stay that much sharper and quicker. If you also eat the right foods in a varied and balanced diet, remembering that the metabolism slows down as we get older, so calorie intake has to be adjusted accordingly, and enjoy a good social life, you will be doing the best you possibly can to ensure good health in your old age.

The motivation for keeping trim and fit can actually be stronger at this stage in your life than ever before. But you may need to learn self-discipline in a way that was not necessary previously. Your day is your own, but you need to organize it to get the best out of it.

One daily fixture you should make a top priority is to take some form of physical exercise for at least 1 hour each day. Walk as much as possible, and investigate the full range of physical activities specially designed for your age group at your local adult education institute (see Chaper 5). Classes are remarkably good value and won't make inroads on a tight budget, if you are living on a pension or fixed income. But they will pay handsome dividends in terms of the way you look and feel.

One form of exercise you might particularly like to consider taking up in retirement is aquarobics: keep fit with a difference – in the water. These exercises, which are suitable for non-swimmers, make use of both the natural support and density resistance of water to tone and strengthen the muscles. They are particularly good for anyone suffering from rheumatism or arthritis, or recovering from a bone fracture, as the buoyancy of the water takes the strain off joints and facilitates movement. Aquarobics classes are often organized at local authority swimming pools. To practise on your own in the water, here are some simple bending and swinging exercises – make sure you do them at a time when the pool is not too busy.

To strengthen back, buttock and thigh muscles:
1 Stand sideways on to the pool wall, holding on with one hand.
2 Standing straight, swing one leg backwards and forwards, keeping the muscles braced.
3 Reverse the position and repeat with the other leg.

1 Face the side of the pool, standing in fairly shallow water, holding on to the side with both hands, feet slightly apart.
2 Rise on tiptoe, bend both knees outward and lower, keeping your back straight and your weight over your feet.
3 Return to standing position on tiptoe, then drop to your heels.

To strengthen hip and inner thigh muscles:
1 Face the pool side and hold on with both hands.
2 Stand on one leg, foot flat. Slowly swing the other leg out to the side, keeping the upper body straight and immobile.
3 Repeat with the other leg.

EIGHT

Diet and the Firm Figure

Exercise, as we have seen again and again throughout this book, is absolutely essential to toning and strengthening muscles, and thereby acquiring a lithe and shapely body. This will happen more quickly, efficiently and effectively if you also follow the right diet. Exercise and diet should ideally be combined in a dual approach to successful figure-firming.

Diet and exercise are truly complementary because not only does one assist the other – the more exercise you take, the more excess fat is used up by the working muscles – but the slimmer your body becomes, the easier and more pleasurable it will be to exercise. And as a more shapely figure emerges, the less you will be tempted to eat the wrong things and destroy all the good that exercising has done for you. For this reason, exercise can actually make you feel less hungry.

Calorie control

We took a look at calories in Chapter 1, where we saw that the energy equation is really very simple:

- to *maintain* your weight at a stable level you need to ensure that you don't consume more calories than you can readily burn up;

- to *lose* weight you need to burn more calories than you consume.

The obvious way to get the energy equation right is to reduce your food intake and step up your physical activity through exercise simultaneously in an integrated programme.

The metabolic rate varies from one individual to another. In the same way, it is not 'fixed' within each individual. The metabolism changes in the course of life – tending to slow down, for example, as we get older – and can be adjusted according to the body's different needs at different times.

So far this book has looked in detail at one side of the energy equation – the different ways to take exercise to your figure's advantage. Now it's time to look at the other side – the diet factor – and immediately some striking similarities in the right approach to both diet and exercise emerge.

Throughout the sections on exercise we have seen how important it is to take exercise *regularly*, to develop an exercise routine tailored to individual requirements and to make it a natural part of your everyday life. Occasional spurts of vigorous exercise don't work to firm your figure – it is steady, consistent exercise that does this.

The same is true of diet. Crash dieting, like sporadic exercise, is useless for genuine, lasting figure control. Instead, what you need is a sensible, balanced eating plan which will work for you in the long term. A crash diet will mean you lose quite a few pounds in the early stages as a rule. But the weight shed is made up of water and glycogen (a form of starch stored in the body to be converted to glucose, for energy, as needed) rather than the excess fat which is what you want to lose. After a crash diet you will all too easily regain the weight you have lost – a very dispiriting experience, guaranteed to make you give up on diet for good. And crash dieting, if undertaken for too long a period, can eventually have an adverse effect on your entire metabolism, upsetting the body's balance.

Just as with exercise, you need to develop an eating plan that will suit you as an individual and fit around the kind of lifestyle you lead. In the same way, too, just as you may have needed to rethink your whole approach to exercise as a prelude to getting your figure fit, you may find you also need to revise the eating habits of a lifetime, to get your figure under dietary control.

We have seen that if exercise is to be effective in figure terms, it must be enjoyable and fun. It is just as important to enjoy what you eat, otherwise you are very unlikely to want to keep to any diet plan in the long term – and this is exactly what you need to do for results. People who 'enjoy their food' and 'love cooking' are very often the ones who need to watch their diet most. If you belong to this category, you will find that it is perfectly possible to eat sensibly and enjoyably, and to cook creatively and interestingly, while keeping your calorie intake low. A good dietary plan, like good exercise, should be a constructive pleasure, not a chore.

Again as with exercise, your mental attitude towards losing weight and keeping slim is of the utmost importance. You need to be really determined, at the same time realizing that you are not setting out to achieve instant results overnight. Both diet and exercise, to be effective in a worthwhile way, are long-term processes, requiring a considerable degree of patience and commitment. If you try to start before you have both these, you are unlikely to succeed in your aims.

In Chapter 2 it was suggested that the first valuable step to take in evolving a figure-firming exercise programme is to give your body an objective appraisal in a 'self-screening' test. In the same way, the best start to adapting to a healthy diet that will help you stay firm for life, is to make a full and frank assessment of your eating habits.

Be really honest with yourself. Do you ever:

- nibble between meals?

- binge if you feel depressed, for 'comfort'?

- help yourself to seconds when you're not really hungry?

- skip proper meals and then indulge your hunger with easy-access junk foods?

- eat too many fatty, sugary foods?

Most people who need to lose weight will probably answer 'yes' to some if not all of these points. So already we have the outline of a figure-firming plan:

- Eat regular meals – 'little and often' is a very useful ground-rule. This means always starting the day with a proper breakfast (see ideas on page 119); not missing lunch, however hectic your day turns out to be – taking a healthy packed lunch to work, for example (see page 126); and trying not to eat too late at night – not only is this bad for your digestion, but there is much less opportunity to shift calories if you go to bed immediately after eating. Eating in this way to satisfy your hunger on a regular basis means that you will be much less inclined to binge.

- However, if you know you are prone to between-meal snacking, and find that habit hard to kick at first, do your figure a favour by keeping a supply of healthy, low-calorie nibbles like celery or carrot sticks ready prepared in the vegetable drawer of the refrigerator. Or pop an apple or satsuma into your pocket or handbag to satisfy any hunger pangs that may occur during the course of the day away from home.

■ Use exercise itself to keep yourself from eating unwisely. For example, many people find their weakest moment is when they come home from work. It is all too tempting to fix yourself a quick cheese sandwich, slice of buttered toast or stiff gin and tonic accompanied by a handful of nuts, to keep yourself going till suppertime. If you can programme yourself to exercise at this time, as suggested in Chapter 2, your figure will benefit, particularly as the muscles are ideally receptive to exercise by this time of the day.

■ Most importantly, cut out the fatty foods, especially those that contain saturated fat, and the sweet, sugary foods high in calories and low in other nutrients. Consult the list of 'No-No Foods' on page 113 and stick to it.

■ Replace these foods with those that provide the necessary balance of complex carbohydrate, fibre, complete protein, and a certain amount of fat, and vitamins and minerals to provide the energy and chemicals from which healthy muscles, bone, blood and body tissue are built.

Fat in the diet

Gram for gram, fat contains over twice as many calories as protein or complex carbohydrate. A certain amount of fat in the diet is necessary, for concentrated energy, but it is the saturated fats, usually of animal origin, that you want to avoid.

Saturated fats are found in dairy products such as butter, milk, cream and cheese, and animal products like lard and suet. Avoid them by:

■ substituting polyunsaturated vegetable margarine or low-fat spread for butter

■ using skimmed or semi-skimmed milk instead of full-fat

109

for pouring on cereal, using in cooking and making drinks, and limiting yourself to about ½ pint/300 ml per day

■ cutting out cream in favour of low-fat yogurt, avoiding the types described as 'thick and creamy'; if you do use cream occasionally, bear in mind that single and soured cream contain 19 per cent fat (and 'half cream' only 12 per cent) compared with 55 per cent in clotted cream, and 48 per cent in double

■ choosing low-fat cheese, especially cottage cheese, for use in salads, sandwiches, etc. rather than full-fat types. Cottage cheese – which you can buy in a variety of appealing flavours, with prawns, with chives, with fresh pineapple, etc. – makes deliciously moist sandwiches with wholemeal bread! So moist in fact, you won't need butter

■ When you eat meat, choose lean cuts, and reduce your fat intake further by trimming off and discarding all visible fat – which includes the skin on chicken

■ In cooking, and for salad dressings, use polyunsaturated vegetable oils, such as sunflower, or monounsaturated, like olive oil, rather than butter or lard

■ Avoid cakes, biscuits, pastries, croissants, pies, chocolate, fudge, toffee, etc., all of which have a high fat content

Sugar in the diet

Don't overload your body with the kind of 'empty' calories you get from foods with a high refined sugar content. You're being really unfair to yourself figure-wise if you indulge in these, as you'll have to work twice as hard to burn off the calories, and these high-calorie foods too often contain little in the way of other nutrients. Think of sweet, sugary foods as real obstacles in your figure firming plan, and resist them accordingly!

■ Cut out sweetened drinks and replace these with unsweetened fruit juice and diet drinks

■ Indulge a craving for something sweet with fresh fruit rather than confectionery – there's an abundance of exciting exotic fruits in the shops to try as alternatives to apples and pears, when you want a change from everyday fruit

■ If you buy canned fruit, make sure it's in natural juice, not sugar syrup

■ Try to cut out sugar in tea and coffee, replacing it with an artificial sweetener if you miss the sweet taste

■ Get into the habit of sweetening plain yogurt or cereal (always avoid cereals with added sugar) with pure clear honey rather than sugar – there are some wonderful perfumed types of honey to choose from

■ If you enjoy baking, try cutting down on the sugar content of cakes, puddings and biscuits by using dried fruits – bananas, dates and apricots as well as raisins, currants and sultanas – instead

■ Get into the habit of checking food value labels carefully to make sure 'hidden sugar' has not been added, and go for products marked 'without added sugar' – it's amazing what a difference this can make.

Further diet tips

As well as cutting down on fat and sugar, and eating as widely as possible from the different nutritional groups, the following may also help to make your figure-firming eating plan easier and more enjoyable:

■ Eat slowly, chewing your food well, to satisfy your appetite more completely, as well as aiding your digestion.

■ Choose a smaller plate from which to eat smaller servings of food, so as not to feel that you are depriving yourself.

■ Aim for attractive presentation. A smaller amount of food that's made to look good can be as satisfying as a larger helping when it appeals to the eye as well as to the taste-buds – take a tip from the masters of nouvelle cuisine here!

■ Although sufficient fluid intake is extremely important for correct body functioning, especially of the kidneys, taking in too much liquid in the course of the day can result in fluid retention, which may often contribute to weight gain. Watch the number of cups of coffee and tea you drink on a daily basis, both at work and at home.

■ And keeping an eye on liquid intake includes alcohol too, of course, as part of any calorie-controlled diet. As a general rule, a simple unit system will keep you within the 'safe' limits. With one unit of alcohol being equivalent to a glass of wine, a measure of spirits, or a half pint of beer, it is recommended that women should not drink more than 14 units a week, and men not more than 21. (In case this sounds like discrimination, the differential is actually based on the fact that women tend to have more fat and less water in their bodies, so that alcohol tends to stay in women's bodies for longer, and in a more concentrated form than in men's.) You can of course adjust the weekly total in terms of daily intake – drinking a glass of wine with your evening meal on weekdays, for example, leaving a total of 9 units, in the case of a woman, to be used up over the weekend, if you are going out to a Saturday night party or Sunday lunch. But drinking less alcohol generally is bound to show in the way you look – and feel!

The no-no foods

Say no to the following, and at one fell swoop you will be removing many of the most common obstacles in food terms to figure-firming success.

- Butter and block margarine

- Cream and all products containing cream, such as cream-based sauces, dressings and mayonnaise, cream soups, ice-cream

- Fried foods, unless a minimum of unsaturated oil is used

- Any food cooked in lard or dripping, such as roast potatoes

- Fatty meats, such as breast of lamb or duck

- Full-fat cheeses, both hard and soft, such as Cheddar and full cream cheese

- Meat products, such as sausages, pâtés and salami (products marked 'low-fat' are permissible)

- Nuts (unless you are vegetarian)

- Crisps

- Avocado pears (wickedly high in calories)

- Biscuits, both sweet and savoury

- Pastries, both sweet and savoury

- Pies

- Puddings

- Confectionery, especially chocolate, toffee, fudge, caramels, butterscotch, Turkish delight, coconut ice

Balancing your diet

Put at its simplest, any low-fat, low-sugar, high-fibre diet combined with regular exercise qualifies as 'calorie-controlled'. Following this type of combined programme should ensure a steady loss of 1-2 lb (0.5-1 kg) a week (acknowledged as the ideal way to lose weight) and certainly will guarantee a slimmer, firmer you.

Some people find the idea of calorie counting helpful and reassuring. Once you have reduced to reach your target weight, and discovered how many calories you need to maintain it (which varies from one individual to another), you are well on the way to retaining that new, firm figure indefinitely.

Others, especially those to whom figures in the sense of sums do not come so easily, may find the calculations involved in calorie-counting offputting. And it is also true that restricting what you eat solely in terms of calories can be misleading. For even if you get your sums absolutely right, and your daily intake spot-on in terms of your energy requirements, you may still not necessarily end up eating the right foods.

Say you have decided to restrict yourself to 1,000 calories a day, for example, you could do this by eating:

1 individual pork pie (420 calories)

4 oz/100 g cashew nuts (610 calories)

but you would be bound to feel very hungry by the end of the day, and no one would begin to suggest that this could possibly represent a balanced diet.

Thus while it is extremely useful to be aware of the calorie values of different foods – which can sometimes otherwise take you by surprise – it is really more advisable to think of your complete diet in terms of how it should be made up from the different food groups, rather than listing individual food items for the calories they contain. In other words, you will be aiming to follow a diet that is as varied, balanced and nutritionally sound as possible.

Now that we have established the importance of cutting back on fat – especially saturated animal fat – and sugar – refined carbohydrate – in the diet, let's look at the more positive side: what you can eat, in quantities that will ensure you never feel hungry, and served in ways that will never leave you feeling bored.

When you are following a diet-and-exercise figure-firming programme, you want to be particularly sure that you are eating the right foods to fuel all of your body's energy requirements, without gaining weight. The ideal energy foods are complex carbohydrates: cereals and grains, legumes and other vegetables, and fruit. These are also valuable sources of dietary fibre and a range of important vitamins and minerals. From this group, which should represent 60 per cent of the energy content of your diet, you will find the following particularly valuable:

- rice, especially brown rice, excellent as a base for main-course dishes like risottos and substantial salads, as well as an accompaniment to curries, kebabs, etc.

- oats, now believed to have special cholesterol-lowering properties, with which you can make sustaining breakfast porridge or muesli, or bake healthy biscuits, and other grains like cracked wheat, delicious in Middle Eastern *tabbouleh*, with masses of chopped parsley and mint, and in other salads.

■ wholemeal flour, which gives goodness and flavour to all kinds of baking. 1-2 oz (25-50 g) wholemeal bread per day is recommended as part of a slimming diet for its nourishing, sustaining qualities.

■ the same is true of wholewheat pasta, especially if served with a fresh vegetable-based sauce, like tomato or spinach. Cooked pasta shapes are also good in salads, tossed in a low-calorie yogurt dressing.

■ pulses – all sorts of peas, beans and lentils, for making colourful salads, hearty casseroles and bakes, dips, pâtés, purées and sauces, and stuffing mixtures.

■ vegetables can be served in virtually unlimited quantity as part of a body-firming diet, and it is worth experimenting to make the most of them. Jacket-baked potatoes, for example, are entirely acceptable slimmers' food, provided they are topped with a swirl of low-fat yogurt sprinkled with chives rather than butter or soured cream. Or they can be made into a complete meal with the addition of tuna and sweetcorn, or cottage cheese and prawns, or baked beans, or grated Edam cheese. Other root vegetables make appetizing casseroles, cooked long and slowly in stock, a little wine and plenty of herbs, or boiled until tender and mashed to a purée, with a little fromage frais added for extra smoothness.

Tender vegetables like French beans, mangetout, broccoli and asparagus cook to perfection in a microwave oven, retaining all their flavour and colour without losing any of their

texture. A variety of vegetables – such as sliced carrots, courgettes and runner beans, and cauliflower broken into florets –
benefit from quick stir-frying in a wok or frying pan with a
minimum of oil, and cooked vegetables as well as assorted
green leaves make splendid salads. 'Fruit vegetables' – tomatoes, sweet peppers and aubergines – are perfect for stuffing
and baking and serving as a complete main course dish.

What is true of vegetables applies equally to fruit too.
You're spoiled for choice for fruit in any well-stocked super-
market, greengrocer or market stall, and there are just as
many ways of cooking and serving fruit, which makes ideal
snacks as well as healthy desserts. Start the day with a fruity
breakfast – mixed with cereal and muesli, or made into a refreshing cocktail or compote. Try cottage or curd cheese
mixed with slices of peach and banana, and fresh strawberries, for lunch, or serve it scooped into pear halves. For a
healthy, non-fattening pudding, try stuffing baked apples
with a mixture of soft fruits – raspberries and redcurrants, for
instance – or dried chopped fruits. Dried apricots, stewed and
puréed, then folded into whisked egg white, make a light and
refreshing fool, and the same principle can be used to freeze
low-calorie sorbets – mango, blackcurrant or passionfruit, instead of ice-cream, which will now be off your list.

The protein foods do not feature as abundantly as the complex carbohydrates in a controlled diet – nutritionists regard
about 15 per cent of total intake as an acceptable protein level
– but they are important because they contain the amino-
acids (substances containing nitrogen) which are vital in the
body's chemistry. Complete protein foods contain all 22 of
the amino acids, including the nine described as 'essential'
because they cannot be manufactured by the body but must
be provided in the diet.

Good sources of protein are eggs, fish, seafood, chicken, lean meat and pulses, all of which may feature in controlled quantities on a slimming diet. Six oz (175 g) per day of fish, chicken or meat would be considered sufficient, plus a serving of a low-fat dairy product, another useful source of protein. It is recommended that the consumption of eggs should be limited to three per week, as egg yolk is high in cholesterol. Pulses are valuable sources of complete protein in a vegetarian diet when combined with grains: lentils with brown rice, for example.

So however much you like to eat, you will find a more than sufficient variety of the right kinds of food on a low-fat, low-sugar, low-fibre body-firming diet, which means that you need never feel that you are making sacrifices, or that you're following a spartan regime.

In the same way, if you enjoy cooking, you will still find that you can develop your skills and add to your repertoire at the same time as watching the calories. Preferred cooking methods for figure-watchers are:

■ *steaming*: ideal for vegetables, fish and shellfish. An expandable steamer which will fit in any size saucepan is a useful piece of kitchen equipment.

■ *grilling*: good for chicken portions, small cuts of meat and fish, and kebabs of fish, meat, vegetables or fruit.

■ *stir-frying*: perfect for cooking vegetables, meat, fish and seafood with a minimum of oil. A wok, kept well-seasoned, is ideal.

■ *dry-frying*: a special heavy ridged pan creates the effect of grilling on top of the hob. Good for cooking steak, lean-mince burgers and chops, as the fat just drains away.

■ *baking*: foil-wrapped meat and fish cooks to perfection without added fat. By the same principle, use roasting bags for joints of meat – no fat or dripping is needed, and the meat cooks to mouthwatering tenderness and succulence.

■ *microwave*: for its brilliance with vegetables alone, a microwave will pay dividends.

■ *pressure-cooking*: as you will be eating lots of vegetables as part of your figure-firming diet, you may find that the pressure-cooker proves invaluable for cooking them in a fraction of the time it normally takes.

7-day figure-firming eating plan

Breakfasts
1 1 oz (25 g) corn or bran flakes with 1 oz (25 g) raspberries, and skimmed or semi-skimmed milk
2 Poached egg on 1 slice wholemeal toast
3 Citrus cocktail (grapefruit, orange and satsuma segments) 2 crispbreads spread with polyunsaturated margarine or low-fat spread
4 Poached or grilled mushrooms on wholemeal toast spread with marmite, garnished with grilled tomato halves
5 1 oz (25 g) muesli and 1 small chopped dessert apple, with skimmed or semi-skimmed milk
6 5 fl oz (150 ml) natural low-fat yogurt with 1 sliced banana
7 1 oz (25 g) porridge, made with skimmed or semi-skimmed milk, with 1 oz (25 g) seedless raisins or stoned prunes

Lunches
1 2 slices wholemeal bread, topped with sliced Edam cheese and tomato; garnished with lettuce and watercress

2 4 starch-reduced crispbreads, spread with 2 oz (50 g) tuna in brine, drained and mashed with 1 teaspoon low-calorie mayonnaise, topped with cucumber slices

3 8 oz (225 g) baked beans in tomato sauce on 1 slice wholemeal bread

4 4 oz (100 g) cottage cheese mixed with fruits of your choice – peach, pear, apricot, kiwi, strawberries, etc. 2 crispbreads

5 Omelette made with 2 eggs

6 Home-made thick mixed vegetable soup with toasted wholemeal croûtons

7 Open smoked salmon sandwiches garnished with mustard and cress and lemon wedges

Suppers

1 6 oz (175 g) chicken joint, grilled with lemon juice and capers served with sweetcorn and broccoli spears

2 4 oz (100 g) lean beef, stir-fried with shredded ginger, bean sprouts, mangetout and sliced spring onions, and served with 2 oz (50 g) rice (cooked weight)

3 6 oz (175 g) white fish, grilled with lemon and capers, served with steamed leeks and boiled potato

4 4 oz (100 g) lamb's liver, grilled as a kebab and served with carrots and Brussels sprouts

5 4 oz (100 g) peeled prawns, curried with mixed vegetables and served on brown rice

6 Wholewheat pasta with tomato and grated courgette sauce, sprinkled with 2 teaspoons grated Parmesan cheese, accompanied by a green salad, with various kinds of readily available leafage

7 Black-eyed bean and mixed vegetable hotpot, served with brown rice.

These suggestions are just a selection of ideas for meals to feature in a figure-firming eating plan. You'll collect many more – from friends, slimming books, health magazines and newspapers, as well as the ones you create for yourself. Collect your tried and tested favourite slimming recipes in a paste-in cuttings book, to which you can keep adding. This way, you will build up a repertoire that proves conclusively that eating right, like exercising right, isn't just good for you and your figure, but creative and fun as well.

Balanced menus

Here is a selection of suggestions for a week's balanced menus as part of a figure-firming plan. For dessert ideas, for either lunch or dinner, see page 123.

Day 1

Breakfast   3 apricots or prunes with 5 fl oz/150 ml natural yogurt

Lunch   1 jacket potato topped with 2 oz (50 g) cottage cheese with chives

Supper   4 oz (100 g) lamb's liver, grilled or fried in a minimum of sunflower oil, with mushrooms, sliced green beans and 2 new potatoes

Day 2

Breakfast   1 slice wholemeal toast topped with 1 oz (25 g) grated Edam cheese and grilled with 1 tomato

Lunch   1 hardboiled egg, sliced, with 1 teaspoon low-calorie mayonnaise, sprinkled with mustard and cress and served with plenty of mixed salad, accompanied by 2 crispbreads or slices of melba toast

Supper   4 oz (100 g) monkfish, marinated in lemon juice and herbs and grilled as a kebab with spring onions and pieces of red pepper, and served with rice

Day 3
Breakfast   4 fl oz (100 ml) freshly squeezed orange juice, 1-2 weetabix with skimmed milk

Lunch   1 wholemeal bap filled with 2 oz (50 g) corned beef, 1 teaspoon of your favourite pickle and lettuce and tomato

Supper   4 oz (100 g) chicken breast, brushed with clear honey and spread with grain mustard, and baked, with broccoli spears and carrots

Day 4
Breakfast   Fresh fruit salad with a variety of fruits in season or compote of stewed fruit, 1 slice wholemeal bread, toasted, with marmite

Lunch   Salad of cooked brown rice, sweetcorn, beetroot and sardines

Supper   4 oz (100 g) beef sausages, grilled, served with steamed cauliflower florets, grilled onion rings and tomato

Day 5
Breakfast   1 baked apple

Lunch   1 wholemeal pitta bread filled with tongue, sliced olives and shredded lettuce

Supper   4 oz (100 g) salmon steak, foil-baked with herbs and cucumber, served with boiled potato and French beans

Day 6

Breakfast Kipper kedgeree
Lunch Celery sticks and 2 oz (50 g) Brie
Supper Baked aubergine stuffed with lean mince, tomato and chickpeas

Day 7

Breakfast 2 rings of fresh pineapple with 2 oz (50 g) curd cheese
Lunch Eggs and cress wholemeal sandwiches
Supper Fillet of lamb, grilled, with diced root vegetables and stir-fried cabbage

Fruity desserts

When you are watching your figure, eating plenty of fresh fruit is the ideal way to satisfy a natural craving for something sweet. Fresh fruit by itself supplements any meal perfectly, as well as making healthy in-between-meal snacks, if you get really hungry.

With the abundance of home-grown and exotic varieties now available through the year, it would be impossible to ever get bored with fruit. Here are some ideas for ways to use fruit in desserts which could be eaten with any of the lunch or supper suggestions on pages 119-121. If you use canned fruit, do make sure it is in natural juice, not sugar syrup.

Stuffed fruits

Apples or pears stuffed with dried or fresh fruit, topped with a teaspoon of clear honey and baked, need no added sugar.

Fruit jellies

Stewed apples, apricots, damsons, etc., puréed and set with

gelatine or agar-agar, make refreshing natural jellies – much nicer than the packet variety.

Fruit kebabs

Pieces of fresh fruit such as pineapple, banana, pear, apple, and hulled strawberries and stoned cherries look and taste good threaded on to wooden skewers, brushed with a mixture of orange juice and honey, and grilled.

Fruit crunch

Any mixed fresh fruit, combined with natural yogurt and muesli, makes a super-quick, appealing dessert.

Melon halves

Small melons, such as ogen or charentais, are delicious filled with soft fruits in season, with a dash of port if liked.

Fruit fools

Gooseberries, raspberries, strawberries, rhubarb or black-berries, puréed and sieved, then folded with natural yogurt and whisked egg white, make light and creamy fools.

Arranged fruit salad

A few pieces of fruit – slices of kiwi, mango and pear, seg-ments of grapefruit and orange, whole raspberries and straw-berries – look most attractive arranged on a pretty serving plate, accompanied by a blackberry or blackcurrant coulis.

Vegetable variety

Vegetables are invaluable sources of complex carbohydrate, fibre and important vitamins and minerals, so play a vital part in a healthy, well-balanced diet. Fortunately they are mostly

low in calories, so you can afford to eat them in virtually unlimited quantity as part of your figure-firming plan. Avoid
tossing vegetables in butter or deep-frying them in oil, and the
results will not only be much healthier, but will taste much
fresher and more natural too.

Every season of the year brings its own special vegetables,
which means they are an excellent way of adding variety to
the diet.

Winter
Vegetable purées are delicious with plainly grilled chops or
roast game birds. They also make a good base for vegetable
terrines and soufflés – broccoli and spinach are very successful
used in this way – or for filling other vegetables: open mushrooms filled with leek purée, for example. A simple but subtly
flavoured mixed root vegetable purée, combining swede,
parsnips, carrots, potato, turnips, mashed smoothly with a
little sunflower margarine and skimmed milk, is a splendid
way of transforming humble vegetables into something really
special.
Winter salads. Root vegetables can also provide the base for
some tasty, nourishing and substantial winter salads: diced
beetroot, with apple, for example, in a yogurt dressing, or
grated carrot, diced celery and sultanas. An interesting variation on coleslaw, an ever-popular winter salad, combines
shredded Brussels sprouts, grated carrot, fresh orange seg-
ments and chopped dates. Pulses, too, are excellent in salads:
try chickpeas with spinach and yogurt, for example.
Vegetable soups and curries: ideal warming fare during the
winter months.
Stuffed vegetables in winter can make a complete meal: baked
potatoes with an endless variety of fillings; baked onions or

125

cabbage leaves with a minced meat stuffing, flavoured with warm spices such as cinnamon or nutmeg.

Vegetable stir-fries: quick stir-frying retains all the nutrients, colour and texture of many different kinds of vegetable – cabbage, leeks, mushrooms, carrots, baby sweetcorn, broccoli spears, cauliflower florets, and so on.

Summer

Salads: leafy green salads are the very essence of summer eating. There is a wonderful choice of salad leaves – several varieties of lettuce, including radicchio and oak-leaved, now becoming almost as familiar as Cos or Webb's Wonder, and rocket, dandelion and tender spinach leaves as well.

Stuffed vegetables: late summer brings a crop of vegetables ideal for stuffing: sweet peppers, big juicy tomatoes, courgettes and aubergines. Other vegetables, rice, pulses and different kinds of meat and seafood can all be featured in stuffing mixtures.

Steamed vegetables: the baby vegetables of early summer benefit greatly colour and texture wise from steaming, and lose none of their goodness either. Sugarpeas, baby carrots, young broad beans, tender asparagus and tiny new potatoes are all at their best when steamed, and like all vegetables will benefit from the addition of chopped fresh herbs in season.

Vegetable canapés: vegetables are not just for everyday eating. You can also use them to lend a sophisticated, low-calorie note to party food: tiny cherry tomatoes, cucumber and celery boats, and miniature button mushrooms filled with hummus or curd cheese, for example.

Packed lunches

When you're busy at work, it's all too easy to skip lunch, but as already seen (page 108), regular meals and not going for long periods without food are essential in a healthy eating plan. Packing your own lunch is a good way of ensuring this, and with a little forethought you can always be sure of a really appetizing and sustaining meal – better than any fast food takeaway or hasty pub lunch – that will satisfy your natural midday hunger and carry you through the rest of the day energetically and efficiently.

Sandwiches: give these extra interest by making them with a variety of breads – wholemeal, granary, rye, pumpernickel; use reduced calorie bread for extra figure-conscious sandwiches; spread with low-fat spread, vegetable margarine or low-calorie mayonnaise. Make sure there is plenty of filling and that this always includes vegetables – not just lettuce, cucumber and tomato, but watercress, sliced red pepper rings, spring onion, beansprouts, grated carrot, sliced olives, asparagus tips, etc. Fruit – banana, dates, apple – is also delicious in sandwiches.

Here are some suggestions for sandwich fillings:

- Eggs, either hardboiled or scrambled

- Cheese, ideally Edam, cottage, curd or Brie

- Meat, especially lean beef, corned beef, meat loaf, lean ham, chicken or turkey without skin, tongue

- Fish, especially sardines, tuna, salmon, prawns, crab, anchovies

Pitta pockets can accommodate copious filling and make a great lunch. Any of the above fillings would be suitable, plus strips of omelette, hummus and other pulses, like mashed red kidney beans.

Salads pack easily into containers. Savoury salads based on rice and pulses make especially sustaining lunches, perhaps with a carton of fresh fruit salad to follow.

Home-made soups can readily become part of a packed lunch routine if·you invest in a wide-necked thermos flask.